AQA Human Health and Physiology

GCSE

Niva Miles

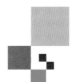

Nelson Thornes

Published in 2009 by:
Nelson Thornes Ltd
Delta Place
27 Bath Road
CHELTENHAM
GL53 7TH
United Kingdom

11 12 13 / 10 9 8 7 6 5 4 3 2

A catalogue record for this book is available from the British Library.

ISBN 978 1 4085 0399 7

Cover photograph by Getty/Jon Feingersh

Illustrations include artwork drawn by GreenGate Publishing

Page make-up by GreenGate Publishing, Kent

Printed in China by 1010 Printing International Ltd

Special acknowledgments

I would like to dedicate this book to Peter, my rock and life support
system, to my lovely children, Bethan, Owain, Sian, Berian and
Elena, granddaughter Rhianna and to my darling mum, Alice.

Niva Miles

Contents

Introduction   4

How Science Works   6

1 Cells and cell processes   10

2 Nutrition   14

3 Digestion   20

4 Blood and the circulation system   26

5 Gas exchange   34

Examination-style questions for Chapters 1–5   37

6 Excretion   46

7 Nervous system, hormones and coordination   50

8 Muscles, bones and movement   60

Examination-style questions for Chapters 6–8   64

9 Human reproduction and birth   70

10 Human growth and development   74

11 Inheritance and genetic engineering   78

12 Pathogens and defence against disease   84

Examination-style questions for Chapters 9–12   91

13 The immune response   96

14 Cancer   100

15 Twenty-first century health   104

16 The controlled assessment   108

Examination-style questions for Chapters 13–16   110

Answers to 'Apply what you know'   116

Glossary   121

Index   124

Nelson Thornes and AQA

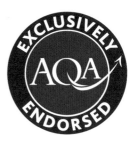

Nelson Thornes has worked in partnership with AQA to make sure that this book offers you the best possible support for your GCSE course. All the content has been approved by the senior examining team at AQA, so you can be sure that it gives you just what you need when you are preparing for your exams.

■ How to use this book

This book covers everything you need for your course.

Learning Objectives

At the beginning of each section or topic you'll find a list of Learning Objectives based on the requirements of the specification, so you can make sure you are covering everything you need to know for the exam.

> **Objectives**
> **Objectives**
> **Objectives**
> **Objectives**
> First objective.
> Second objective.

AQA Examiner's Tips

Don't forget to look at the AQA Examiner's Tips throughout the book to help you with your study and prepare for your exam.

> **AQA Examiner's tip**
>
> Don't forget to look at the AQA Examiner's Tips throughout the book to help you with your study and prepare for your exam.

AQA Examination-style Questions

These offer opportunities to practise doing questions in the style that you can expect in your exam so that you can be fully prepared on the day.

AQA examination questions are reproduced by permission of the Assessment and Qualifications Alliance.

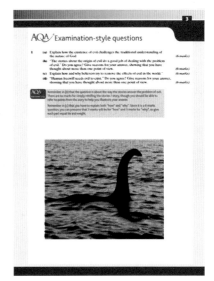

Visit www.nelsonthornes.com/aqagcse for more information.

This student book contains everything you need to know for the AQA Human Health and Physiology GCSE, and also should help you to apply your knowledge to new situations when answering exam questions. The press is full of medically related articles which can be fascinating, informative or just plain gory. There are also many sources of information about the foods we eat and our lifestyle choices. So how can we separate out the facts from the current fads and fashions in diet and treatments?

The Human Health and Physiology guide will help you to understand:

- how the body works
- how we can keep healthy
- how good science is investigated and reported
- some of the language health scientists use.

If you have the opportunity to do the practical work, you will be encouraged to think like a scientist; this is covered in **How Science Works** examples throughout the chapters within this book. As you work through this course you will be encouraged to think about the role of health professionals within society; this is covered in the Scientists@work sections in each chapter.

The How Science Works chapter (pages 6–9) is a summary of the way scientists work so do not be tempted to learn it off by heart before you find out more information about the body, but do keep referring back to this chapter as you progress through the course.

The following features will help you to focus on key points and to avoid common mistakes:

Learning Objectives – you should be able to answer these questions. If you can't, review the content until it's clear.

Examiner's Tips – avoid common mistakes and gain extra marks. Remember, knowing the bare facts is just the starting point. You must understand how the facts link together and be able to apply them to new situations to gain maximum marks in exams.

How Science Works – examples of some of the coursework topics and applications of How Science Works.

Did You Know – some of the more unusual but relevant facts.

Hint – short tips to help you think about the science of Human Health and Physiology.

Scientists@work – information about how people use science in their work life. Human Health and Physiology is an applied science and you should be able to apply what you learn to new situations.

Find Out – short tasks to help you to broaden your knowledge.

Foul Facts – medical facts on the gory side.

Key Terms – are blue in colour where they first appear. Definitions of these terms can be found in the glossary on page 121.

Apply What You Know – test yourself and try to apply your knowledge in new situations before attempting the Exam Style questions.

Sitting Higher Tier – the essential extra knowledge for those intending to sit the HT paper. You can miss this out if you are sitting Foundation Tier. Learning Objectives or questions that cover Higher Tier material are presented in a dark blue colour.

I have been privileged to teach hundreds of students of all ages and many of them have become nurses, doctors, physiotherapists, hospital technicians or research scientists to name but a few of their careers. I hope that some of you, who use this guide to Human Health and Physiology, will be encouraged to continue your studies and eventually join the thousands of health workers or scientists in a wide variety of worthwhile and satisfying jobs.

Niva Miles

How Science Works

Fundamental ideas

There are many skills which contribute to making someone a good scientist, but the key starting point is an understanding of what is meant by **scientific evidence**.

Good evidence is both **valid** and **reliable**. Valid **data** must be relevant to the question and reliable in that it can be repeated by another scientist.

If someone tells you that she bought a crystal to heal her headaches because the man in the shop said 'It works for 90% of my customers', as a scientist you would wonder 'How does he know this? Has he checked with everyone who bought the crystal? How many people bought crystals for this purpose? Did he compare them with people who did not buy crystals?' In other words is his evidence based on scientific **fact** or on **hearsay** and is the shopkeeper likely to be **biased**? Could your friend *prove* that the crystal cured her headache?

The shopkeeper's data is not likely to be valid or reliable.

In the health professions, there are many people who work in a scientific way to collect reliable evidence. But what is the starting point?

Observation

The starting point for many investigations results from an **observation** which triggers a question in the scientist's mind. In this book you will find out how significant observations led to medical breakthroughs:

- Jenner noticed that milkmaids contracted cowpox but not smallpox (see page 98).
- Fleming realised that a fungus was killing bacteria on a Petri dish (see page 88).

Both asked the question 'Why?' and designed **investigations** to gather evidence.

Jenner may have thought:

- 'Something in the cowpox protects the milkmaids' – this idea is his **hypothesis**.
- 'If I infect someone with cowpox they will never contract smallpox' – this suggestion is a **prediction**.
- 'How can I test this?' – this question leads to an investigation.

The observations made during an investigation may support the hypothesis, but if not they could lead to a new idea.

Designing an investigation

Generally the simpler the design the more likely you are to have a clear outcome.

Investigations should be based on the principles of a **fair test**.

Objectives

What is the difference between 'fact' and 'opinion'?

How are observations used to form hypotheses?

How is society involved in science?

What are the limitations of scientific evidence?

Find out ...

- What is meant by valid and reliable evidence?
- What are variables?
- What is a fair test?
- What is the importance of accurate measurements?
- How is data presented?
- How is data used to draw conclusions?

Suppose you want to find out if temperature affects the rate of a reaction:

- only change the **temperature**.
- other things, e.g. volumes, must stay the same – they have to be controlled, so we call them **control variables**.

Investigations test the effect of the **independent** variable, what you change, on the **dependent** variable, the result that you measure. In our example:

- Temperature is the independent variable.
- The time it takes to react is the dependent variable.

Making measurements

When designing the investigation it is necessary to decide the **range** of values and the **intervals** between them for the independent variable:

- Temperature range could be 0°C–50°C or 25°C–75°C.
- Intervals could be every 5 or 10 degrees.

Doing a **trial run** can help to determine these values as well as the number of **repeats** needed and whether or not the instruments are sensitive enough and give consistent readings.

If a measurement is **accurate** it is close to the **true value**.

An instrument which measures to two decimal places is more **precise** than one where the readings are in whole numbers. But be warned! If there is a flaw in the experiment the precise readings may not be accurate. Inaccuracy can occur if the control variables are not controlled, or due to human **error**. To increase reliability, measurements should be **repeated** several times.

Presenting data

While doing an investigation, the easiest way to record raw data is on a **table**:

- Column 1 is used for the independent variable, e.g. temperature.
- Column 2 is used for the dependent variable, e.g. time.

Prepare the table before doing the experiments and fill it in immediately a measurement is made.

In this example the range is 25–75°C; the intervals are 10°C.

The experiment is carried out three times.

Temperature (°C) [independent variable]	Time (minutes) [dependent variable]		
	1	2	3
25			
35			
45			
55			
65			
75			

AQA *Examiner's tip*

Make sure you know the difference between control, independent and dependent variables.

Practical activity

Using humans in investigations

It can be very difficult to control variables in humans. Sometimes age, gender, mass, levels of fitness, whether the person smokes or drinks alcohol can have effects which are not easy to control but can be monitored.

Once the results have been collected they must be analysed and decisions made about the best way to present them, so you can look for **trends** and draw **conclusions**. It might be necessary to simplify the data by calculating the average of your repeats (the **mean**).

Before doing this, it is important to identify any numbers which are too far from the mean. These are called **anomalous** results.

For example, times of 3 + 3.5 + 2.5 give a mean of 3 minutes.

With times of 3, 6 and 2.5 you might decide that 6 does not fit the pattern. You could:

- Do the experiment again to check the time.
- Ignore the '6' in your calculation.

The best way to present results will depend on the independent variable. Use:

- A **line** graph when the variable is **continuous** – it can have any numerical value. Temperature is a continuous variable.
- A **bar chart** for presenting things that can have labels, e.g. eye colour. Values described by labels are called **categoric**. A categoric variable which increases in whole numbers is called a **discrete** variable.
- A **scatter graph** to compare two sets of data, such as the relationship between birth mass of babies and the number of cigarettes smoked by the mother.
- A **pie chart** to represent parts of the whole, e.g. a food analyst could illustrate the food components of a meal in this way.

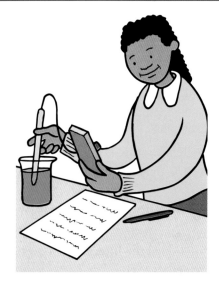

Identifying patterns and relationships in data

The line graph or bar chart will show the relationship between the independent and dependent variables.

Relationships may be:

- **linear** – a straight line
- **directly proportional** – a straight line that starts in the origin
- a **curve**.

Drawing a line, or curve, of best fit can help to make the relationship clear and will show up anomalies in the trends.

The relationship between variables will allow you to draw a conclusion, but how can you be absolutely sure it is reliable and valid?

Extra evidence can be obtained by:

- Checking your results using a different method.
- Asking other people if they can **reproduce** your results.
- Comparing your data with secondary sources, e.g. scientific text books, the internet.

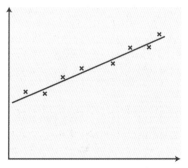

A linear relationship

In scientific research this 'peer evaluation' is a very important part of validating research results before publication.

In medicine, research depends on obtaining data from observation and experiment. This is referred to as 'empirical data'. The data may support the original idea but may also indicate that there are flaws in the suggestion. In this case the scientist has to think of a better explanation

Using the 'crystals cure headaches' hypothesis, reliable data could confirm it or prove it to be wrong. A new hypothesis might be 'if a person sits and relaxes for 60 minutes the headache will disappear' which starts off a whole, new investigation.

Societal aspects of scientific evidence

In this book you will learn how many scientists have been involved in medical research. Scientists have developed new drugs, e.g. insulin and antibiotics, or life saving equipment, and society has benefited as a result. Other advancements such as stem cell and embryo research have been more controversial because they involve ethical and social issues.

Scientists may say 'We can do this', but society may argue 'Should we do this? Can the money be spent in a better way? What impact will it have on the environment?'

Nobody would argue that having new drugs to cure cancer is a bad thing, but recently it has been found that some of these drugs enter the water supply. How might this affect healthy people? Will other scientists be able to solve the problem?

Another problem for the general public is knowing if they can trust what they read. Almost everyday the newspapers carry reports of a new 'superfood' to reduce the risk of cancer, or a diet claiming rapid weight loss if you follow it. If the claims are made by producers of the food or diet product, they may be exaggerated or biased. If possible we should always look for the scientific evidence to back these claims.

Limitations of scientific evidence

Humans are so varied that it can be difficult to control variables in investigations involving them. When thalidomide was developed as a sleeping drug it had not been properly tested for use with pregnant women who used it to prevent morning sickness. It took some time for a **causal link** to be made between the drug and limb abnormalities of babies born to these mothers due to **insufficient evidence** from the initial research.

The role of a scientist is to make new discoveries. The role of society, which includes scientists, is to keep asking 'What should we do with this knowledge?'

Did you know ???????

Over two thousand years ago, Chinese warriors who survived being struck by arrows in war observed that, while they were injured, previous disease and pain in other parts of their body was reduced in intensity and even miraculously cured. This observation is thought to have started investigations into the use of acupuncture.

AQA Examiner's tip

You should be able to 'Apply what you know' about How Science Works in both the written, Unit 1, papers and the ISAs in Unit 2.

1.1 Cell structure, organisation and cellular respiration

Cells – the basic facts

The human body is made up of millions of **cells**. Most human cells contain the same structures:

Cell surface membrane – controls the movement of materials in and out of the cell.

Nucleus – contains our genetic material and controls the activities of the cell.

Cytoplasm – in which most of the chemical reactions take place.

Cheek cells are thin and flat to act as a lining in your mouth. Other cells are specialised to perform a particular function.

Cytologists are scientists who study the structure and function of cells. They need to know how normal cells look and behave so that they can recognise abnormal cells. A **cytotechnologist** prepares slides of cells, e.g. from cervical smears, which can be viewed under the microscope. These cells will be examined either by a specialist technician or a pathologist, who can identify the presence of abnormal cells that may become cancerous.

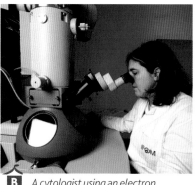

B *A cytologist using an electron microscope*

Find out ...

Examine some cells using a light microscope or 'bioviewer', or find images on the internet, to find out:

- why egg cells are large and have a lot of cytoplasm
- why sperm cells have tails
- why red blood cells lose their nucleus and are packed full of haemoglobin
- why nerve cells have membranes with long threads.

Sitting higher tier

Using electron microscopes, which can magnify the cell more than 100 000 times, cytologists have identified more structures in the cytoplasm. These include:

- ■ **Ribosomes** – to produce proteins such as enzymes, insulin and haemoglobin.
- ■ **Mitochondria** – to release energy in aerobic respiration.

Objectives

What are cells made of?

How is cell structure related to its function?

How are cells organised into bigger body parts?

How do cells get energy?

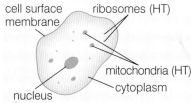
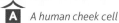

cell surface membrane — ribosomes (HT)

mitochondria (HT)
cytoplasm

nucleus

A *A human cheek cell*

Did you know ???????

One of the most amazing facts in human biology is that a tiny ball of identical cells gradually changes into many different types of cell and eventually forms you. What's more, all the cells are in the correct place!

AQA Examiner's tips

- ■ Learn the relationships between cells, tissues, organs and systems.
- ■ Make sure you know the basic structure of the cell.
- ■ Make sure you can label a diagram of a cell and give the function of each part.
- ■ Note that aerobic respiration takes place in the mitochondria.
- ■ Learn the word equations for respiration.

Cell organisation

A **tissue** is a group of cells with similar structure and function, e.g. muscle tissue, nerve tissue.

Organs contain several tissues to perform a particular function. The arm is an organ containing many tissues, e.g. muscle, bone, blood, nerve.

Systems are groups of organs which perform a particular function, e.g. **digestive** system to digest and absorb food, **skeletal** system to support other organs, **excretory** system to remove waste materials. Some organs can be in more than one system, e.g. the pancreas is part of the **endocrine** (glands) system and the digestive system.

Cellular respiration

Cells need **energy**, **nutrients** (food materials) and **oxygen** to function efficiently.

Respiration is the release of energy from food molecules. Stored **glycogen** and fats are the main energy supplies in cells and these are converted to **glucose** which is used in respiration. All living cells respire, because the body needs energy for building large molecules from small ones, for growth, movement and keeping warm.

Most energy is released from the glucose when oxygen is available to the cell. The process is referred to as **aerobic respiration**. Carbon dioxide is produced by the cells during aerobic respiration and must be removed from the body. Water is also produced.

This word equation sums up the process of aerobic respiration:

glucose + oxygen → carbon dioxide + water + **energy**

During vigorous physical exercise your body may not be able to provide enough oxygen to the muscle cells. The cells start to carry out **anaerobic respiration** (no oxygen) which releases a limited amount of energy and a chemical called **lactic acid**. Lactic acid causes muscle fatigue and cramp.

This word equation sums up anaerobic respiration:

glucose → lactic acid + energy

Apply what you know

1 List all the specialised cells mentioned so far in this chapter.

2 What are the main functions of each of these cells in the body?

3 Cells join to form tissues, organs and systems. Link the cells in your list to examples of these structures.

4 Suggest an advantage and a disadvantage of anaerobic respiration.

5 Which two cells from question 1 use energy for movement?

Groups of cells can be grown, by cytologists, in the laboratory. This is called **tissue culture**. Each type of tissue must be treated differently, but all cells have basic requirements.

6 What must the cytologist supply to cells so that they grow and multiply well? Explain your answer.

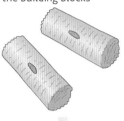

cells:
the building blocks

tissue:
similar cells working together in the same way

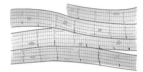

muscle tissue is made of muscle cells that contract and relax together

organ:
groups of tissues working together

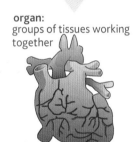

your heart is made of muscle tissue. It pumps blood around your body

system:
a group of organs working together

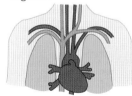

your heart and blood vessels make up your circulatory system.

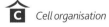   Cell organisation

Foul facts

Lactic acid may cause the burning sensation *during* anaerobic exercise. But the soreness the day after is from tiny muscle tears and inflammation from damaging the muscles.

1.2 | Cell processes

Diffusion and osmosis

Cell membranes are made so that materials can move in and out of the cell.

Molecules (e.g. glucose and oxygen) or **ions** (e.g. sodium ion and chloride) move from the outside into cells and between cells. Glucose and other nutrients enter the body via the digestive system, while oxygen reaches body cells through the lungs. Waste molecules such as carbon dioxide leave the cells and must be removed from the body.

Remember that cell membranes act as a barrier. Only certain substances are allowed in or out of the cell. We say that the membrane is **partially permeable**.

Molecules and ions move between cells by the process of **diffusion**. If there is a lot of oxygen outside a cell it will diffuse into the cell. This occurs because molecules move from an area of high concentration to an area of low concentration.

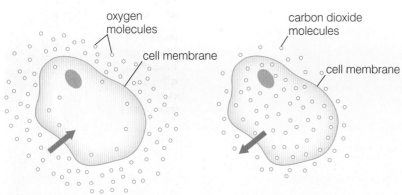

oxygen molecules

cell membrane

carbon dioxide molecules

cell membrane

 Diffusion

Water also diffuses across the partially permeable cell membrane. We refer to this process as **osmosis**. Water moves from an area of high water concentration to an area of low water concentration. If red blood cells are placed in pure water they will burst because water will keep diffusing into the cell. If the red blood cells were placed in a very salty solution water would diffuse out of the cells and they would shrink.

Substances which dissolve in water are called **solutes**. It is important that the body regulates the water and dissolved substances in the blood plasma. This is called the **solute–water balance** (see Chapter 6).

(see Chapter 6)

Objectives

How do materials move in and out of cells?

What is meant by 'diffusion' and 'osmosis'?

What are enzymes and what affects their activity?

Did you know ??????

It is dangerous if even a small amount of sea water gets into your lungs. The salt draws water from the lung cells by osmosis. The water fills up the air spaces. This is called 'secondary drowning'. People saved from the sea should always be checked out by a doctor.

Scientists@work

Health scientists need to learn the language of human physiology so that they can communicate with one another. By learning common words and terms, you will know what other scientists mean. Key words are highlighted in the text.

Enzymes

Cells also need **enzymes**. Cells malfunction when an enzyme is missing or is not working correctly. This can lead to ill health and conditions such as cystic fibrosis (see page 79).

Enzymes are large molecules of protein. Chemical reactions in the cell are controlled by at least one enzyme. Enzymes are a type of **catalyst**, which means they speed up chemical reactions in both building-up and breaking-down processes. Some enzymes can put together small molecules to make larger ones, e.g. during growth of cells. Other enzymes break down large molecules into smaller ones, e.g. during digestion.

Human enzymes work best at about 37°C, our average body temperature. Each enzyme also works best at a particular pH, e.g. the enzymes in the mouth are in alkaline conditions but those in the stomach are in acid. Even slight variations in temperature and pH will change the rate of enzyme activity, but in extreme conditions the enzyme stops working because the protein changes shape – it has been **denatured**. When an egg is heated up, the liquid albumen (a protein) goes solid because the protein is denatured.

Many of the cell processes can be investigated in a school laboratory. You will probably carry out at least one investigation with enzymes. So make sure you know what conditions affect enzyme activity!

How science works

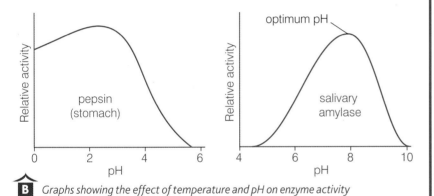

B   Graphs showing the effect of temperature and pH on enzyme activity

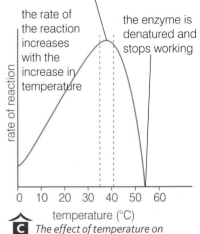

optimum temperature
– this is when the reaction works as fast as possible

the rate of the reaction increases with the increase in temperature

the enzyme is denatured and stops working

C   The effect of temperature on enzyme activity

Apply what you know

Glycogen is insoluble, but is made from large numbers of soluble glucose molecules which are linked together.

1   What type of chemical will join the glucose molecules together quickly?

2   What is the advantage of storing glucose in an insoluble form?

3   Muscle cells and sperm cells have large glycogen stores. Explain why.

4   What type of chemical will break down the glycogen and change it back to glucose?

AQA **Examiner's tip**

■ Remember that osmosis is the diffusion of water.

■ Enzymes are denatured by high temperatures and extremes of pH.

■ Enzymes are proteins so they are produced by the ribosomes.

2 Nutrition

2.1 Nutrition and a balanced diet

What did you eat yesterday? Do you think it was a healthy diet?

Human cells need a range of nutrients (food materials) for healthy growth and development. These nutrients should form part of our normal balanced diet. But what is meant by 'balanced'?

We need to eat foods containing **carbohydrate**, **protein**, **lipids** (fat), **vitamins**, **minerals**, water and **fibre**.

A balanced diet

Dieticians have worked out how much we need of each of these seven food types. This is called the **recommended daily amount** (RDA). But the RDA will vary according to your age, gender and lifestyle. Your dietary requirements will also change during periods of rapid growth, during pregnancy or increased (and decreased!) physical exercise. A doctor may tell a patient to change their diet to control disorders such as diabetes, high blood pressure and heart disease.

So a balanced diet is one which contains all the right nutrients in the right amounts.

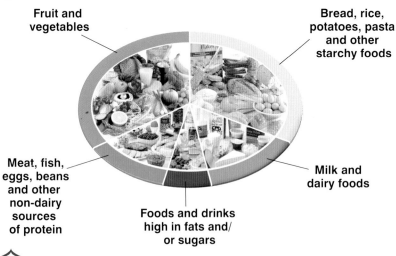

Fruit and vegetables

Bread, rice, potatoes, pasta and other starchy foods

Meat, fish, eggs, beans and other non-dairy sources of protein

Foods and drinks high in fats and/ or sugars

Milk and dairy foods

 A *The components of a balanced diet*

In addition to providing building materials for cells, our diet needs to supply enough energy for movement, chemical reactions, growing and keeping us warm.

Most of our energy is provided by carbohydrate, protein and lipid, so they make up the bulk of our diet.

We also need a wide range of vitamins and minerals, but fortunately you only have to learn about a few of these.

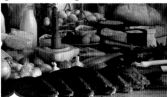

C *The main examples of nutrients you have to know about, rich sources of each one and their function*

Name of nutrient	Rich source	Function
Carbohydrates		Carbohydrates are converted to glucose, which is used in respiration to release energy
sucrose	Refined sugar in sweets and puddings	Surplus sugar is converted to glycogen and stored in cells
glucose and fructose	Sugars in fruit	
lactose	Milk	
starch	Potatoes, rice and grain products	
Protein	Meat, fish	Repairing body tissues, growth of cells Used to make human protein such as enzymes, haemoglobin and antibodies
Lipid (fat)	Butter, oils and lard	Energy store Making cell membranes Covering organs, e.g. kidney, to protect them Provides essential fatty acids
Vitamin A	A fat-soluble vitamin found in cheese, eggs, oily fish and liver	Helps maintain the health of skin Strengthens the immune system Helps vision in dim light
Vitamin D	A fat-soluble vitamin found in oily fish, milk and eggs Also produced in skin cells when exposed to sunlight	Helps the absorption of calcium, which is important for strengthening teeth and bones
Vitamin C (ascorbic acid)	A water-soluble vitamin found in oranges, kiwi fruit, peppers, Brussels sprouts, broccoli	Promotes a healthy immune system Helps wounds heal Helps iron absorption Maintains connective tissue
Calcium	Found in milk, cheese, cabbage, broccoli, okra, soya beans	Needed to strengthen teeth and bones, for muscle contraction, for blood clotting
Iron	Found in liver, meat, beans, nuts, dried apricots, dark green leafy vegetables	Needed to make haemoglobin Also important for many cell reactions
Sodium chloride	These ions are found together as common salt. There are low levels in all our foods, but high levels in processed foods	Sodium and chloride are needed to keep the fluid balance in the body
Fibre	Cereals containing bran. Wholegrain rice, wholemeal bread	Not digested, but adds bulk to food. Absorbs poisons
Water	Water! Any drinks and most food	A medium for chemical reactions, transporting substances and removing excretory substances. Used to cool the body by evaporation

What do I eat?

Nutritionists and dieticians have produced data to help us to choose our foods wisely so that we eat a balanced diet with the correct energy intake. If an adult wants to stay the same weight, the energy intake must balance the energy use. Surplus energy will be stored in the body in fat.

It helps to know that carbohydrate contains 16 kJ/g (kilojoules of energy per gram of food), protein 17 kJ/g and fat 37 kJ/g.

This means that you could eat 100 g of carbohydrate and still have a lower energy intake than if you ate 50 g of fat.

Fibre, although not strictly a nutrient because we do not digest it, is a very important component of our diet. Foods that contain fibre make us feel full, and then we do not over-eat the less healthy options such as fat. Fibre holds on to fat and reduces fat absorption by the body. Fibre also holds onto some toxins, protects us from being constipated and helps to prevent bowel cancer.

Malnutrition

A person can suffer from **malnutrition** if they have:

- too much or too little food,
- too much or too little of one of the nutrients, such as iron or a vitamin. This means that you could have the correct amount of energy but still be malnourished.

Starvation is one form of malnutrition and means the person does not have enough energy for their daily needs, or for growth and repair.

D *Some examples of the causes and consequences of malnutrition*

Cause	Consequence
Not enough food	Lose weight → **anorexia** (dangerously under weight) / starvation → death
Too much energy-containing food, especially fat	Obesity (dangerously overweight) → heart disease, **diabetes**
Too much salt	High blood pressure → heart disease → heart attack
Too much sugar	Obesity → **diabetes**
Too much vitamin A	Stored in liver → becomes toxic
Too little vitamin A	Poor growth. Poor night vision. Weakened immune system
Too little vitamin C	Poor wound healing, bleeding gums, weakened immune system, breakdown of connective tissue → **scurvy**
	Poor iron absorption → **anaemia**
Too little vitamin D	Less calcium absorption → softer bones → **rickets**
Too little calcium	Softer bones and teeth. Poor blood clotting
Too little iron	Less haemoglobin produced → less oxygen carried to cells → less respiration → less energy released → person is tired (anaemia)

Dieting

Dieticians will tell you that the only way to lose weight healthily is to eat a balanced diet, decrease energy intake and increase exercise. The safe, and sustainable, level of weight loss is about 1 kg (2 lb) a week. This allows all the chemical balances in the body to adjust. Diets which have one food in the title are likely to be a 'fad' and difficult to maintain.

If you are eating a balanced diet, you do not need to take dietary supplements, such as multi-vitamin tablets and minerals. But a doctor may suggest a supplement if they suspect a person is suffering from a deficiency disease such as anaemia. Some foods, such as cereals, have supplements added to them. You should think about the issues raised from adding vitamins, minerals, salt, sugar and fat to processed foods.

Did you know ???????

The Food Standards Agency has eight tips for eating well:

- Base your meals on starchy foods.
- Eat lots of fruit and vegetables.
- Eat more fish.
- Cut down on saturated fat (animal fat) and sugar.
- Try to eat less salt – no more than 6 g a day for an adult.
- Get active and try to be a healthy weight.
- Drink plenty of water.
- Don't skip breakfast.

Did you know ???????

The essential fatty acids, omega-3 and -6 must be taken in our diet. We usually have too much omega-6 and too little omega-3. Despite eating a lot of oily fish, Eskimos have little heart disease. This is because the omega-3 in the fish oils actually protects the heart. Do you eat enough oily fish? Try to find out more about these fatty acids.

AQA **Examiner's tip**

You could be asked about other vitamins or minerals, but you would be supplied with the data, so don't be put off!

Did you know ???????

Increase the number of colours on your plate to increase the range of vital nutrients. Brown is better than white.

AQA **Examiner's tip**

Learn *why* lack of a nutrient causes a deficiency disease. It is not usually enough to name the disease.

The Miracle Cabbage Soup Diet

Cut the Carbs!

Woman turns orange on carrot diet

Eat grapefruit & lose weight

I lost stones by eating tomatoes

E *A lot is written in the press about diets and nutrients*

Apply what you know

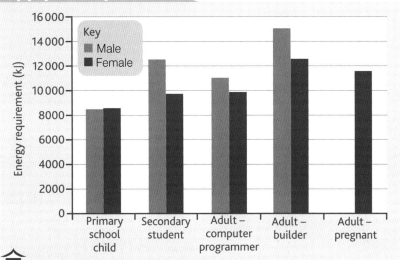

F *Energy requirements of different people*

Look at the graph:

1 How many kilojoules a day should you be aiming for? Remember that these are average figures.

2 What could increase a computer programmer's energy needs?

3 Young children have relatively high energy needs. Why?

4 Why do pregnant women require so much energy?

5 Compare the two plates of food:

a How could you make the fry-up healthier?

b Why is the second meal healthier?

c Which meal contains the most fibre?

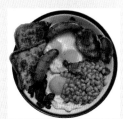

6 Many sailors died from scurvy before the eighteenth century. What was lacking in the sailors' diet?

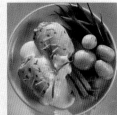

7 The symptoms of scurvy include: dry and splitting hair, gingivitis (inflammation of the gums), bleeding gums, rough or dry skin, decreased wound healing rate, easy bruising, nosebleeds, weakened tooth enamel, swollen and painful joints, anaemia, decreased ability to fight infection, possible weight gain because of slowed metabolism.

Which of these symptoms are likely to be the cause of death?

Foul facts

A man died in the UK in 2008 from drinking too much water over 2 days! The excess water diluted his body fluids, increased his blood pressure and eventually caused him to have a heart attack.

Did you know ??????

Myth

You must drink 8 glasses of water a day.

Truth The amount of water you need to drink depends on how much you sweat, how much salty food you eat and other factors too. It is important to have enough water to prevent dehydration. Feeling thirsty is a good indicator. All drinks supply water.

Hint

Eating is a good way to revise!

Analyse each plate of food you eat. Ask yourself :

'Which food types am I eating?'

'Why does my body need it?'

Then check against the nutrients table.

Picture those plates of food you analysed if stuck on a diet question.

Foul facts

Hundreds of sailors died of scurvy before the eighteenth century. They were not eating fresh foods containing vitamin C. Fortunately scurvy is quite rare now.

Midwives advise pregnant women to avoid eating liver because of the high levels of vitamin A (which can become toxic). This means they need to obtain vitamin D and iron from other sources. Some pregnant women may be prescribed iron supplements.

Scientists@work

If we cooked all our meals from fresh ingredients we could control what goes into them. Realistically we have to buy some food in packets and tins and many people buy ready-made meals. How do we know whether or not the packaged food is healthy?

By law, manufacturers have to put accurate dietary information on their labels.

Here are some examples, but look at some more in your store cupboard.

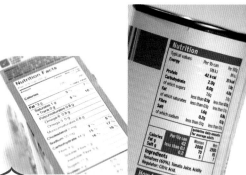
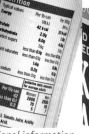
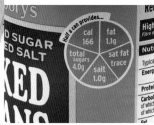

A   *Food packaging showing nutritional information*

The list of ingredients will tell you exactly what is in the packet or tin. The **nutritional information** is usually in a table – this tells you what is in 100 g of the food and may also give the amount per serving.

If you want to compare the fat content of a tin of baked beans and a breakfast cereal, the 100 g column will give a direct comparison. You also need the amount per serving, because you may eat more or less than 100 g.

Food analysts, including nutritionists, use a range of techniques to identify the contents of natural and processed foods.

They need to ensure that there is accurate nutritional information on food labels about the content of the main food groups and the amount of energy, so that customers can judge if the food is healthy for them. Many processed foods contain high levels of sugar, salt or saturated fat, which should be avoided by those trying to reduce the risk of diabetes, high blood pressure or heart disease.

Practical activity

Food tests

In the school laboratory it is possible to test foods for a variety of components. Most of the tests involve a colour change in the reagent. Food scientists will use more complex and precise tests to produce accurate data on food labels.

The table shows which reagents are used in schools and the colour changes if the food component is present.

Objectives

What information is on food labels?

What are the chemical tests for starch, glucose, protein and vitamin C?

How much energy is in a sample of food?

Hint

Every time you open a tin or packet, read the label to familiarise yourself with the data. Try to explain the nutrient information to someone else.

Hint

Remember that your teacher may assess your practical skills in any practical session for the practical skills assessment (**PSA**) and you could have an investigative skills assignment (**ISA**) based on food tests.

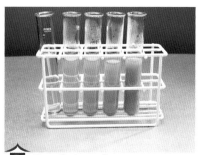

B   *Benedict's test for sugars*

C Colour changes wih reagents for food testing

Food component	Reagent	Colour change
Reducing sugar, e.g. glucose	Boil with Benedict's reagent	Clear blue to cloudy orange
Starch	Iodine in potassium iodide solution	Brown to dark blue/black
Protein	Biuret reagent	Blue to lilac
Vitamin C	DCPIP	Blue to colourless

You can also find out how much energy is in food.

The principle of this experiment is that a piece of food is burned and used to heat water in a boiling tube. The higher the temperature rise, the greater the energy content. The energy can be calculated by using the following equation:

$$\text{energy content (J/g)} = \frac{\text{volume of water} \times \text{temperature rise} \times 4.2\text{J}}{\text{weight of food (g)}}$$

If you do this investigation, you will find that your value is very low compared with the food label. This is because a lot of energy would be 'lost' during the investigation. Food analysts use specialised equipment to reduce heat lost to the atmosphere when they calculate energy content of food.

Apply what you know

Typical values	Barry's Best Beans		Harry's Healthy Beans		Sally's Salmon	
	Amount per 100 g	Amount per serving (200 g)	Amount per 100 g	Amount per serving (220 g)	Amount per 100 g	Amount per serving (110 g)
Energy	310 kJ	620 kJ	300 kJ	660 kJ	700 kJ	770 kJ
Protein	4.9 g	9.8 g	4.4 g	9.68 g	25 g	27.5 g
Carbohydrate	12.9 g	25.8 g	12.0 g	26.4 g	Trace	Trace
(of which sugars)	(5.0 g)	(10 g)	(3.5 g)	(7.7 g)		
Fat	0.2 g	0.4 g	0.5 g	1.1 g	8.5 g	9.35 g
of which saturates	Trace	Trace	0.1 g	0.22 g	1.5 g	1.65 g
polyunsaturates					1.7 g	1.87 g
of which omega-3					1.2 g	1.32 g
Fibre	3.8 g	7.6 g	3.8 g	8.36 g	Trace	Trace
Sodium	0.3 g	0.6 g	0.1 g	0.22 g	0.5 g	0.55 g

1 Compare the data taken from the beans and salmon food labels. Which:

a bean contains the most energy per 100 g?

b bean has the most energy per serving?

c food has the most protein per 100 g?

d food contains the most sugar or salt per serving?

e food contains omega-3 fatty acids?

f is healthier, Barry's Best Beans or Harry's Healthy Beans? Why is it healthier?

3.1 Physical and chemical breakdown of food

■ Physical breakdown of food

Before we can digest our food efficiently, the large pieces of food must be broken down into tiny particles. This process **increases the surface area** of the food.

Most of the physical breakdown occurs in the mouth, by the teeth. Fat is also broken down physically into droplets by bile in the small intestine.

■ Chemical breakdown of food

Starch, protein and fat are large insoluble molecules. These have to be broken down by **enzymes** to turn them into smaller, soluble molecules which can pass across cell membranes into the bloodstream.

The three main groups of digestive enzymes are named after the type of food they digest:

- **Carbohydrases** digest carbohydrates.
- **Proteases** digest proteins.
- **Lipases** digest lipids (fats).

Objectives

How is food broken down to make it soluble?

What are the functions of teeth and saliva?

a **protein molecule** is made up of many different amino acids

protease breaks down protein molecules

amino acids

a **starch molecule** is made up of many glucose molecules

carbohydrase breaks down carbohydrate molecules

glucose

a **fat molecule** is made up of fatty acid and glycerol molecules

fatty acid — glycerol

lipase breaks down fat molecules

fatty acids

glycerol

A *Molecules are chemically broken down by enzymes*

Dentists are health professionals who advise on tooth care, but also repair the damage caused by poor diet and poor tooth cleaning. Dental hygienists support the work of dentists by removing tartar from teeth.

Plaque is a sticky layer, containing bacteria, which forms on your teeth. If you do not brush or floss it away it, the plaque hardens and forms tartar or calculus (see Photo **B**).

Dental hygienists remove the tartar by scraping it away with a special instrument. If you don't have a regular dental check-up your dentist cannot prevent damage to your teeth and gums.

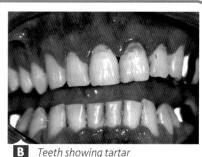

B *Teeth showing tartar*

Teeth

We have four types of teeth:

- incisors
- pre-molars
- canines
- molars.

They all have the same basic structure, but different shapes.

The enamel is very hard but can dissolve in acid. If too much erosion (decay) occurs the softer, sensitive, dentine may also be damaged, eventually exposing the pulp. Then you get toothache, because the nerve endings are stimulated.

Saliva is an alkaline liquid produced by the **salivary glands**. It helps to neutralise acids in the mouth.

Here are ways you can reduce the effect of acid:

- Do not eat or drink too much acidic food or drink such as fresh citrus fruit or cola.
- Drink water with acidic foods to wash away the sugar and acid.
- Clean your teeth before meals to remove bacteria or afterwards to remove food particles. Bacteria digest sugar in the food and produce acid.

Saliva is also important in dissolving soluble food and, without saliva, food would be hard to swallow. Saliva also contains the enzyme **amylase** which starts the digestion of starch.

If you eat a cream cracker you bite it with the incisor teeth. Saliva is added to the cracker in your mouth and you chew it with the molar and pre-molar teeth to crush it into small particles. Your tongue mixes the cracker particles with saliva and amylase changes starch in the cracker to sugar. The cracker is then ready to swallow.

Swallowing is a reflex action which occurs when your tongue pushes the food to the back of your mouth. A flap called the **epiglottis** covers the opening of the windpipe as you swallow. The slimy **mucus** in saliva helps the food to slip down into the **oesophagus** (the gullet).

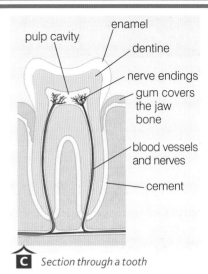

C *Section through a tooth*

labels: pulp cavity, enamel, dentine, nerve endings, gum covers the jaw bone, blood vessels and nerves, cement

Find out ...

The British Dental Association has a good website. Use it to learn about tooth decay.

Did you know ?????

The Guinness Book of World Records states that, in 2005, Ambrose Mendy consumed three cream crackers in 34.78 seconds. No mean feat, as the crackers soak up saliva very quickly. Try it!

Practical activity

What happens when we bathe teeth in acid?

If your teacher can obtain some 'teeth' – place them in different acid concentrations or different types of acid food, e.g. orange juice, vinegar. What happens to the enamel?

A good way to simulate teeth is to use clean chicken bones. Bones and teeth both contain calcium salts. Leave the bones in acid overnight – they should go soft. **Remember to wear eye protection**.

Practical activity

Eating to learn

Bite into a piece of bread or a cream cracker. Which teeth did you use?

Now chew the bread or cracker slowly and record what is happening. Which teeth do you use? Is anything else in your mouth? Try not to swallow the bread or cracker. What is happening to the dry food? Does it taste sweet?

Apply what you know

1. Dentists advise that cleaning children's teeth straight after giving them fruit may do more harm than good. The success of health campaigners to increase fruit in the diet has led to higher levels of tooth decay where parents are also conscientious about brushing after every meal. Can you explain why?

2. Why do you get toothache when decay reaches the dentine and pulp?

The gut

The gut (or alimentary canal) is one long tube, but each organ has a particular job to do. The salivary glands, **pancreas** and gut lining contain specialised cells which produce the digestive enzymes. The **digestive juices** containing these enzymes pass into the gut where they are mixed up with the food. To help the mixing process, and to push the food along, the muscular walls of the gut contract and relax, this process is called **peristalsis**.

The squeezing action of peristalsis brings the enzymes into contact with the food molecules. Once the enzymes and food are well mixed the conditions must be just right for the enzymes to work. Each enzyme has a particular pH in which it works best (see page 13).

A *Summary of enzyme action in the digestive system*

Region where digestion takes place	Name of enzyme	Where is the enzyme produced?	What does the enzyme do?
Mouth	Amylase – a carbohydrase	Salivary glands	starch → sugar
Stomach	Protease	Cells in stomach lining	Starts to change: protein → amino acids
Small intestine	Carbohydrases	Pancreas +	carbohydrates → simple sugars
	Proteases	Cells in lining of small intestine	protein → amino acids
	Lipase		fats → fatty acids and glycerol

pH and enzymes

Each digestive enzyme works best in a small range of pH. The pH ranges from slightly alkaline in the mouth to very acid in the stomach (see page 13). This means that amylase stops working when the food reaches the stomach. Stomach protease works well in acid but is denatured in the small intestine.

Objectives

How is food digested?

What are the functions of the organs in the digestive system?

What happens to digested food?

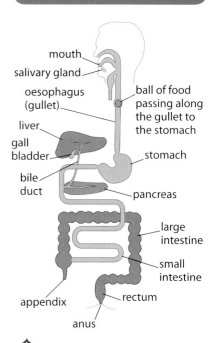

mouth
salivary gland
oesophagus (gullet)
liver
gall bladder
bile duct
appendix

ball of food passing along the gullet to the stomach
stomach
pancreas
large intestine
small intestine
rectum
anus

B *The human digestive system is 9 m long in adults*

Practical activity

Activity to simulate peristalsis

You will need:

1 balloon, flour and water.

Make a thick dough. Spoon some dough into the opening of the balloon. Squeeze the dough along the balloon. Where do you press?

Pour some water into the balloon. Is the dough still lumpy? Now hold the open end of the balloon tight and squeeze the contents with your other hand. What happens to the lumpy dough?

The stomach

The stomach acts as a bag to hold the food for a few hours. This allows us to have three meals a day instead of eating every half hour. The acid in the stomach not only activates a protease but also kills microbes which are swallowed with the food. The cells of the stomach are protected from the acid by a layer of mucus.

Small intestine

The acidic food is squeezed out of the stomach a bit at a time. It enters the small intestine and must be neutralised. **Bile,** which is made by the **liver** and stored in the **gall bladder,** enters the small intestine via the **bile duct.** Bile contains several chemicals. The **alkaline salts** in the bile neutralise the stomach acid so that enzymes from the **pancreas** (see Table **A**) can work properly.

The bile is also important in breaking fat into small droplets. This is called **emulsification.** Bile acts on fat like the detergent you add to washing up.

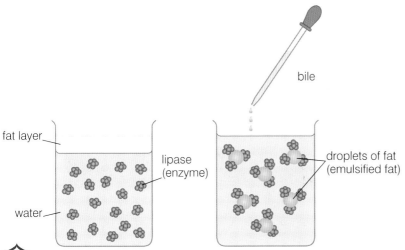

C Bile breaks fat up into small droplets. This increases the surface area so that the lipase can reach more fat molecules

By the time the pancreas and small intestine enzymes have acted on the food, most of the large insoluble carbohydrates, proteins and lipids should be broken down to simple sugars, amino acids, fatty acids and glycerol. The intestine will contain a very watery solution of these molecules as well as soluble vitamins and minerals. Insoluble fibre will also be in the intestine.

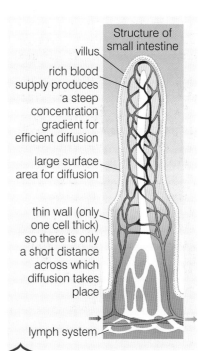

Structure of small intestine

villus

rich blood supply produces a steep concentration gradient for efficient diffusion

large surface area for diffusion

thin wall (only one cell thick) so there is only a short distance across which diffusion takes place

lymph system

D Section through a villus in the small intestine

Absorption

The small intestine is designed to absorb the soluble food. The inner surface of this 6 m tube is covered in tiny finger-like projections called **villi,** which increase the surface area by about nine times.

Each villus has a very thin wall, only one cell thick, which allows soluble food molecules to diffuse through to the capillaries underneath. The blood carries the food away to the liver so a concentration gradient is maintained.

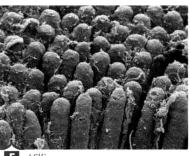

E Villi

The cells on the surface of the villi are covered in minute **microvilli** which are folds of the cell surface membrane. The microvilli increase the surface area of the intestine a further 20 times.

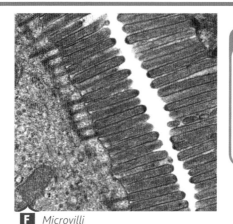
F *Microvilli*

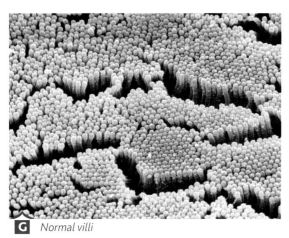
G *Normal villi*

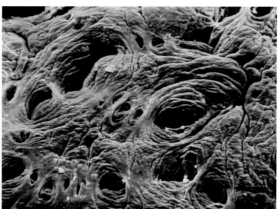
H *Villi of person with coeliac disease*

What happens to the absorbed food?

Following absorption the food is **assimilated**. Glucose, fatty acids and glycerol can be used for energy release. Surplus glucose is taken up by the liver and muscle cells and stored as glycogen or converted into fat. Some fatty acids and glycerol are used to build cell membranes and to make some hormones. Surplus lipids are stored in fat cells. The amino acids are used to make protein for building cells or for making enzymes and haemoglobin.

Sitting higher tier

Excess amino acids cannot be stored. They are carried to the liver and broken down by a process called **deamination**. During deamination, ammonia is produced. The liver converts the toxic ammonia into **urea** which is excreted in the urine.

The large intestine

By the time your meal has reached the large intestine, all the soluble nutrient molecules should have been absorbed. The gut still contains a lot of water (think of all the 'juices' that have been added), indigestible fibre and millions of bacteria. Most of the water is reabsorbed by the large intestine and the faeces which remain are **egested**.

Sitting higher tier

Cystic fibrosis

Cystic fibrosis (CF) is an inherited disorder (see page 81) that causes the body to produce thick, sticky mucus. The mucus blocks the pancreatic duct so that digestive enzymes cannot reach the duodenum from the pancreas. The mucus also covers the surface of the villi, preventing the efficient absorption of nutrients.

Coeliac disease

Coeliac disease is a condition which is triggered by a protein, gluten, found in cereals. The gluten causes the immune system to attack the villi, which reduces the surface area of the villi available for absorbing food.

Practical activity

Make a model gut using dialysis tubing

This experiment combines food tests, enzyme activity and diffusion through membranes.

Set up three 'guts': one containing starch solution, one containing starch and amylase, one containing starch and boiled amylase. Suspend the model guts in separate boiling tubes of water for 30 minutes.

After 30 minutes, test the water around the model guts for starch and reducing sugar using the iodine and Benedict's tests.

[Starch will not be found in the water because it is too large to diffuse through the gut. Sugar will only be found in Tube 2 because the starch has been digested and the sugar is small enough to diffuse through the tubing.]

Apply what you know

1. Do we need to digest glucose?

2. In the model gut experiment, name the enzyme, substrate and product, independent variable, dependent variable and two controlled variables.

3. Why do cystic fibrosis and coeliac disease reduce the digestion and absorption of nutrients?

Did you know ???????

The number of bacteria in the large intestine can exceed the number of body cells you have!

Hint

Remember that **bile** is made in the **liver**.

Foul facts

Ulcers can develop in the stomach if the acid reaches the cells and damages them. But most ulcers are caused by a bacterium, *Helicobacter pylori*, which can survive and multiply in the stomach acid.

Did you know ???????

Drinks normally go down the oesophagus by gravity. Astronauts in negligible gravity need the power of peristalsis to move their drinks down. Peristalsis can move drinks up to the stomach if you are turned upside down!

4 Blood and the circulation system

4.1 Blood

Blood is vital to human life because it carries materials to every cell in the body and takes away waste products. Blood is actually a tissue but the **blood cells** are suspended in a liquid, the **plasma.**

There are three main types of blood cell: red cells, white cells and platelets.

Red blood cells are packed with **haemoglobin**, which is the oxygen-carrying molecule of the blood. As red blood cells develop from stem cells they lose their nucleus and become flattened and disc shaped. Without a nucleus there is more room for haemoglobin and the shape gives a larger surface area for efficient diffusion of oxygen into the cell.

Oxygen is picked up in the lungs and carried to all the body cells:

oxygen + haemoglobin → oxyhaemoglobin in red blood cells

White blood cells protect the body against disease. They are part of the immune system and there are two main types. The **lymphocytes** produce antibodies and the **phagocytes** engulf pathogens such as disease causing bacteria (see Chapter 13). They are much larger than red cells and there are fewer of them.

Platelets are cell fragments which are needed for blood **clotting** when you cut yourself. Clots prevent the loss of more blood and the entry of pathogens that might cause infection.

Sitting higher tier

If a blood vessel is damaged, the platelets release enzymes setting off a chain of reactions. The final reaction involves a soluble blood protein, **fibrinogen**, which is changed by an enzyme to insoluble **fibrin**. The network of fibres produced traps blood cells and forms the clot.

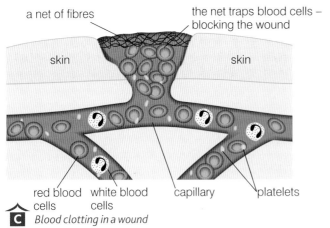

a net of fibres

the net traps blood cells – blocking the wound

skin   skin

red blood cells   white blood cells   capillary   platelets

C Blood clotting in a wound

Plasma is the body's main transport medium, containing dissolved glucose, amino acids, fatty acids, glycerol, vitamins, minerals, carbon dioxide, urea and many other chemicals such as hormones.

Objectives

Why is blood vital to life?

What are the jobs of blood cells?

Why do we need to know our blood group?

platelet

red blood cell   white blood cell

 A Three types of blood cell

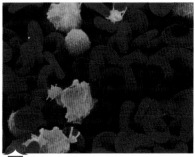

B Human blood cells

Find out ...

Adult humans have about 5 million red blood cells per cubic millimetre of blood. Can you work out how many there are in the 5 litres of blood in the body? What products are obtained from blood? How are they stored?

Learn more about the work of the National Blood Service at: www. blood.co.uk

The National Blood Service of England and Wales collects, screens, processes and delivers blood and blood products to hospitals for use in surgery and other treatments. Many scientists are involved in ensuring that the blood is safe to give to patients. Some determine the blood type, or check that the blood is free from transmissible disease. Others separate the blood components in order to make blood products, for use in specific treatments, and package them appropriately e.g. plasma is frozen. Specialists in radiation treat some products for procedures such as bone marrow transplants.

Most patients only need one component. Red blood cells may be given to someone with anaemia, factor VIII to a haemophiliac whose blood does not clot without it, but whole blood is also used where the patient has bled significantly.

Research scientists in the National Blood Service look for new ways to use blood products and improve safety.

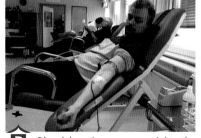

D Blood donations are essential to the National Blood Service

Blood groups

If a patient is to receive a **transfusion** of whole blood or red blood cells they must be of the correct blood group. There are four main types of human blood: **A**, **B**, **AB** and **O**. In the UK about 44 % of the population are group O, 42% are A, 10% are B and 4% are AB. Group O blood can be given to patients with all four blood groups and is referred to as the **universal donor**. If the wrong blood type is given to a patient, the red blood cells will stick together (they **clump**) which can prove fatal.

Sitting higher tier

Lack of haemoglobin causes **anaemia**. This may be due to iron deficiency, or a factor like internal bleeding or excessive blood loss in menstruation. Low haemoglobin means less oxygen is carried to the cells; there is less aerobic respiration and less energy available so the person becomes tired easily.

Sitting higher tier

Blood groups are determined by molecules called **antigens**. These are found on the cell membranes of red blood cells. The immune system produces antibodies which attack foreign antigens causing clumping.

In group O blood the cells do not have antigens, so the blood of the person receiving a donation of O will not have antibodies to attack it. The O cells will not clump.

If AB blood was given to a person with group O, the A and B antibodies would attack the A and B antigens causing the donated blood cells to clump. The combinations of antibodies and antigens can be shown on a compatibility table.

Blood group	Antigens	Antibodies	Can donate blood to	Can receive blood from
AB	A and B	None	AB	AB, A, B, O
A	A	B	A and AB	A and O
B	B	A	B and AB	B and O
O	None	A and B	AB, A, B, O	O

Burns victims dehydrate rapidly because the skin has been damaged. Water evaporates from the exposed body cells. In such cases the doctor will give the patient a plasma transfusion to replace the water, maintain the fluid balance in the body and provide other essential blood components.

Apply what you know

1 Make a list of all the things which might be in the blood.

2 What are the advantages of red blood cells losing their nucleus and having a disc shape?

3 The blood clotting process only starts if a vessel is damaged. Why is it important that clots do not form inside the blood vessels?

4 Before DNA testing, forensic scientists could use blood found at a crime scene to identify suspects. How can blood type be identified? It was often possible to eliminate people from enquiries but not to definitely convict them. Why is this?

4.2 Circulation

Most of the cells in your body are a long way from the gut or the lungs. The body needs an efficient method to move materials from these organs to the cells. Other things must be transported too:

- waste products are transported from the cells for removal by organs such as the lungs or kidney
- hormones are transported from glands to other organs where they are needed
- heat is transmitted from working muscles to the whole body.

The **blood** is the transport medium and it flows in **blood vessels**. The organ which keeps blood circulating is the **heart**, the body's pump.

▉ The circulatory system

Humans have a **double circulation**. Blood from the right-hand side of the heart is carried to the lungs where the red blood cells collect oxygen. This **oxygenated** blood returns to the left-hand side of the heart and is then pumped to the rest of the body. The cells take up the oxygen and the **deoxygenated** blood eventually returns to the right-hand side of the heart.

Arteries carry blood away from the heart. **Veins** carry blood to the heart. **Capillaries** are tiny blood vessels which lie very close to the body cells.

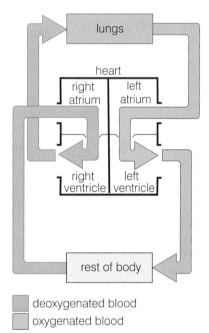

deoxygenated blood
oxygenated blood

A *The double circulation system*

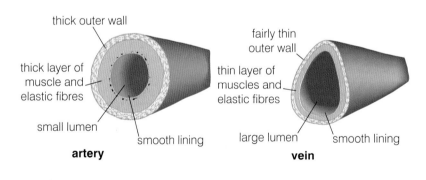

thick outer wall

thick layer of muscle and elastic fibres

small lumen

smooth lining

artery

fairly thin outer wall

thin layer of muscles and elastic fibres

large lumen

smooth lining

vein

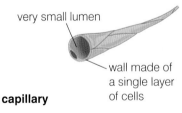

very small lumen

wall made of a single layer of cells

capillary

B *Arteries, veins and capillaries*

Arteries

Blood is forced into the arteries from the heart. The high pressure causes the elastic walls to stretch and then they spring back, helping the blood to move along. This action is felt as a **pulse** at your wrist or other pulse points.

Veins

The walls of veins are thin and less elastic. The blood in veins is forced back to the heart as the body muscles press against the veins. When you walk about the leg muscles press against the leg veins, moving the blood uphill! The veins have valves inside to prevent backflow.

Capillaries

The walls of capillaries are very thin. This allows soluble molecules to diffuse across the wall and enter the cells. Soluble waste from the cells diffuses in the opposite direction. The capillary network provides a massive **exchange surface** between the blood and body cells.

The heart

If you place your left fist in the centre of your chest it will give you an idea of the position of your heart which is slightly tipped towards the left side.

Look at the diagram of the heart and you will notice that it is actually two muscular pumps joined down the middle. The right pump forces blood to the lungs. The left pump forces blood around the body.

Blood enters the heart from the veins and passes into the upper chambers, the **atria**. This starts a cycle of muscle contractions. Both pumps contract together. As each **atrium** contracts the blood is pushed against **valves** which are forced open and the blood enters the **ventricles**. These are thick walled chambers so when the muscles contract they force the blood into the **arteries**.

While the ventricles contract the atria relax, allowing blood to enter from the veins again. Valves stop backflow from the ventricles to the atria. Other valves stop the blood going back into the heart from the arteries when the ventricles relax.

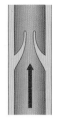 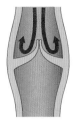

valves open to let the blood flow toward the heart

valves close to stop blood flowing backwards

 Valve action in the veins

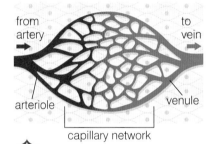

from artery

to vein

arteriole

venule

capillary network

D *Capillary network around the body cells*

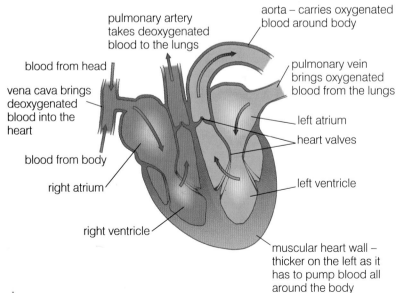

pulmonary artery takes deoxygenated blood to the lungs

aorta – carries oxygenated blood around body

blood from head

pulmonary vein brings oxygenated blood from the lungs

vena cava brings deoxygenated blood into the heart

left atrium

heart valves

blood from body

right atrium

left ventricle

right ventricle

muscular heart wall – thicker on the left as it has to pump blood all around the body

 The heart

Sitting higher tier

Blood pressure

The blood is at its highest pressure as it is forced out of the ventricles. The large arteries help to maintain the pressure as they pulse, but as the blood branches into smaller vessels (arterioles) the pressure decreases until it reaches the capillaries. Blood flows more slowly through the capillaries, allowing time for exchange of food and oxygen.

The graph shows the fall in pressure through the blood system.

Key
aorta   – main artery
arterioles – branches of arteries
venules   – small veins
vena cava   – main vein

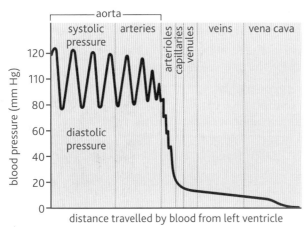

F   *Blood pressure in the circulatory system*

You may be asked to explain changes in the content of the plasma as the blood circulates. For example, the carbon dioxide concentration and heat will increase close to active muscle cells due to aerobic respiration; urea increases as blood passes through the liver; the hormone insulin will enter the blood when the glucose levels are high. You will come across these and other examples as you study the various body systems.

Heart muscle

Heart (cardiac) muscle needs a constant supply of glucose and oxygen for aerobic respiration to supply the energy needed for the heart to beat. If one of the **coronary arteries** is blocked by a blood clot, the blood will not flow to the cardiac muscles and the person will suffer a **heart attack**. One of the main causes of a blockage is the narrowing of the internal space of the arteries as a result of fatty deposits on the walls, called **atheroma.** Atheroma may develop as a consequence of high cholesterol in the diet.

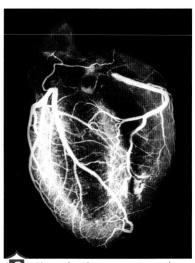

G   *Heart showing coronary vessels*

Symptoms of narrowed blood vessels can be the chest pain felt from a condition called **angina**. Blood clots may form on the roughened artery walls and move to the coronary vessels supplying the heart muscle, causing a heart attack.

■ Strokes

Blood clots can also form in the brain. If brain cells do not receive oxygen they will die causing brain damage. The resulting stroke symptoms may be quite mild, temporary speech loss and numbness, or severe physical disability. 80% of strokes are caused by clots. The other 20% are due to bleeding in the brain from burst blood vessels.

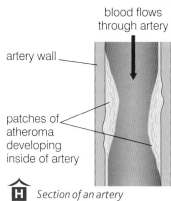

blood flows through artery

artery wall

patches of atheroma developing inside of artery

H   *Section of an artery*

> *Scientists@work*
>
> Much preventive medicine depends on maintaining a healthy circulation and monitoring people at risk of heart attacks. **Cardiac physiologists** record heart activity to compile scientific data for doctors, and may implant and evaluate **pacemakers**. **Cardiographers** help them by using monitors to record the electrical activity of the heart. Following heart surgery or a stroke, a physiotherapist may use massage to stimulate the blood flow and will advise the patient on exercises to maintain a healthy circulation.

Sitting higher tier

Keeping pace

The natural resting heart rate is controlled by a group of cells in the right atrium called the pacemaker. Sometimes, due to ageing or heart disease the heart may miss a beat, slow down or beat irregularly. Scientists have developed an artificial pacemaker which fits under the skin in the chest. It is an electrical pulse generator attached to the heart by one, two or three wire leads, which stimulates the heart to beat regularly. The leads are placed into the appropriate heart chambers depending on the patient's particular heart problem. The pacemaker, weighing 20–50 g, contains a battery and an electronic circuit and is placed between the skin and chest muscle.

Did you know ??????

The process of building up atheroma is called atherosclerosis. **Risk factors** for atherosclerosis are:

- smoking
- high blood pressure
- high blood cholesterol
- low levels of activity
- diabetes
- obesity
- family history.

Scientists@work

Born on 1 April 1578, William Harvey worked out how the blood circulates around the body.

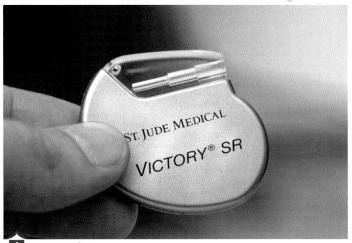

I   *A pacemaker*

Foul facts

GTN is used to treat angina, often as a spray under the tongue. This is the same chemical used in dynamite as an explosive!

Heart to heart

Most of the time we take our heart for granted, but when it does fail it has a devastating effect on our lives. Occasionally, the damage to the heart is so severe that surgeons decide the patient needs a **heart transplant**. The first surgeon to conduct a heart transplant on a human was **Christiaan Barnard** in 1967. The patient had been very ill but survived for 18 days before dying from a lung infection. Barnard became instantly famous worldwide and he was credited with being a great medical pioneer. Since then many successful heart transplants have taken place, over 2000 of them performed by **Sir Magdi Yacoub** in London.

Professor Yacoub continues to head groundbreaking research to find new ways of treating patients with heart disease and valve failure, because there are never enough donors for those who need transplants.

When patients undergo a heart transplant they are attached to a **'heart–lung'** machine while their own heart is removed and the new one inserted. The machine has a pump and an oxygenation system in order to circulate blood to all the body cells during the operation. The blood must also be kept warm and free from contamination.

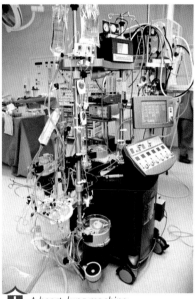
J *A heart-lung machine*

The organ care system

Researchers have developed the world's first portable system, which allows a new type of transplant called **living organ transplant**. This new technology, called an 'organ care system' is designed to maintain the organs in a warm, functioning state outside of the body.

1 The donor heart is placed in a sterile chamber, which keeps the organ at body temperature.

2 Blood from the heart donor is oxygenated, combined with nutrients and pumped into the heart through the aorta, keeping it beating.

3 Blood flows through the heart, leaving via the pulmonary artery.

aorta

pulmonary artery

K *Organ care system*
© Transmedics, Inc.

Sitting higher tier

Modern techniques to treat heart disease may involve the use of mechanical hearts fitted to the patient. The blood is diverted through the mechanical heart and, together with the use of drugs, allows the patient's own heart to recover sufficiently to improve their quality of life.

Narrowing or leaking heart valves may also be replaced by donor human valves, pig or cow valves or artificial valves. Patients who receive artificial valves need to take anticoagulants daily to reduce the risk of blood clots.

Research scientists, including Professor Yacoub's team, have been attempting to grow **stem cells** to produce heart valves and possibly hearts! (See page 83 for stem cells.)

When donor hearts become available they have to be tissue typed. Certain donor antigens must be as close as possible to those of the recipient. Following a transplant the patient is given immunosuppressant drugs to combat the body's immune system. This stops rejection of the organ.

Practical activity 🔍

Investigate exercise and pulse rate

This may form part of an ISA or PSA. You will need to decide what type of exercise to do, what you are measuring and which variables you have to control.

Is it easy to control human variables?

Apply what you know

Physiotherapists give help and advice to patients after heart attacks and strokes. They give guidance on exercises, lifestyle changes and relaxation techniques to aid recovery.

1 Why is it important to exercise?

2 What changes in lifestyle might the physiotherapist suggest?

3 What changes in diet would a dietician suggest for someone with heart disease?

4 Pacemakers are programmed by computers to match a patient's needs, but most pacemakers have sensors to detect body movement and will speed up the rate of impulses when the person is active. Why is this important?

5 a Suggest some of the ethical problems faced by Christiaan Barnard.
    b Suggest some of the practical problems faced by Sir Magdi Yacoub.

6 List the pros and cons of modern methods of treating heart disease. Don't forget ethical, social and economical issues.

5.1 Gas Exchange

Aerobic respiration in our cells is the most important process to maintain life. The oxygen required is obtained from the air and the carbon dioxide produced must be removed from the body. The **lungs** are the vital organs which allow this **gas exchange** to take place.

Objectives

How does air get into the lungs?

How are alveoli adapted for efficient gas exchange?

How is breathing coordinated?

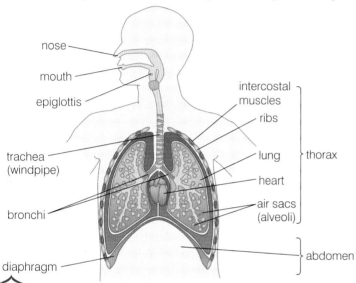

A *Diagram of the breathing system and the pathway of the air into the lungs*

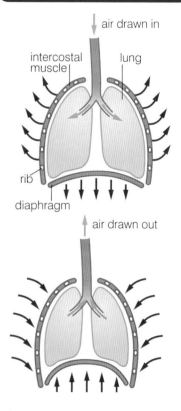

Sit upright and breathe in deeply through your nose. You will notice that your chest rises. The **intercostal muscles** between the **ribs** contract to pull up the rib cage. At the same time your **diaphragm** contracts and flattens. This increases the **volume** of the thorax and decreases the internal **pressure** so that air is drawn in.

As air is inhaled it is cleaned and warmed. In the nose large particles are filtered out by hairs and mucus. Tiny particles and bacteria are trapped by mucus lining the air tubes. **Cilia** are like tiny hairs on the surface cells of the air tubes, which beat to move this mucus up to the throat to be swallowed or coughed out. Cigarette smoke destroys cilia so the mucus accumulates in the lungs and the smoker must cough to remove it.

B *The process of breathing*

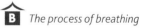

The clean air passes through the bronchial tree, which spreads the air from the **trachea** over a much wider surface, and enters millions of tiny air sacs called **alveoli**. Each alveolus is adapted for efficient gas exchange.

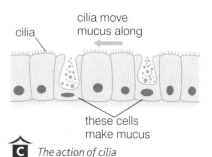

C *The action of cilia*

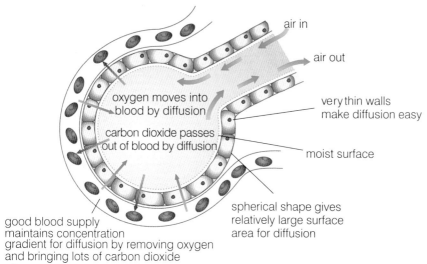

air in

air out

oxygen moves into blood by diffusion

carbon dioxide passes out of blood by diffusion

very thin walls make diffusion easy

moist surface

spherical shape gives relatively large surface area for diffusion

good blood supply maintains concentration gradient for diffusion by removing oxygen and bringing lots of carbon dioxide

D *An alveolus*

Scientists@work

All cells need a good supply of oxygen for respiration. All health professionals, including paramedics, need to understand how oxygen reaches the cells from the air and the consequences of lack of oxygen, such as damage to the brain.

Faced with two casualties, one of whom is screaming, the other very quiet, a paramedic will realise that the noisy patient has clear **A**irways, is **B**reathing and has a **C**irculation (the A, B, C of first aid). The quiet casualty needs to be assessed quickly for these signs, in case they need help to breathe.

Pulmonary technicians measure lung volumes. They use monitors to record how much air the person normally breathes in and out (the **tidal volume**) and the maximum amount of air they can breathe in (the **vital capacity**). A decrease in capacity may indicate lung disease.

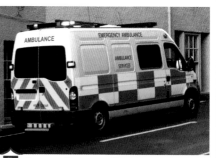

E *Paramedics responding to an emergency*

Sitting higher tier

Breathing is coordinated by the respiratory centre in the **brain**. Carbon dioxide makes the blood more acidic. This is detected by pH **receptors**, which signal the brain to increase the breathing rate. When the pH rises (is less acidic) the breathing rate will reduce. Mouth-to-mouth resuscitation depends on delivering expired air to the casualty. The increased carbon dioxide is detected by the brain which stimulates the breathing muscles to contract.

Practical activity 🔍

You should now be able to work out the relationship between heart rate, breathing rate and exercise. This could be an ISA or PSA.

Apply what you know

1 What happens when you breathe out? List the sequence of events.

2 Try gently pressing on your windpipe (trachea) – what can you feel? What is the function of the cartilage rings on the bronchial tree?

3 Why does oxygen enter the blood and carbon dioxide leave? Use your knowledge of diffusion and concentration gradients to work this out.

4 What features make the alveolus efficient?

5 Some smokers and people who work in dusty environments may suffer from emphysema, a lung disease where the alveolus walls weaken and collapse. The person will gasp for breath and be very tired. Can you explain why?

6 Do a short spell of vigorous exercise. Stop and think about your breathing. What changes do you notice?

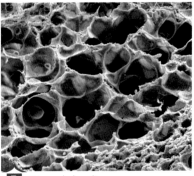

F *Normal alveoli*

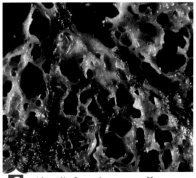

G *Alveoli of emphysema sufferer*

Scientists@work

Scientists in Swansea are developing a portable artificial lung for patients with conditions such as cystic fibrosis and emphysema. Eventually they hope to produce a device which can be inserted into the chest. The ultimate goal would be to make an artificial lung which may prevent the need for a lung transplant.

The patient will be connected to the device and their blood pumped through it (see Diagram **H**). The blood would be in close contact with a flow of air. Gas exchange will occur inside the device, which must be made of materials that do not stimulate the blood to clot. The oxygenated blood returns to the patient's bloodstream.

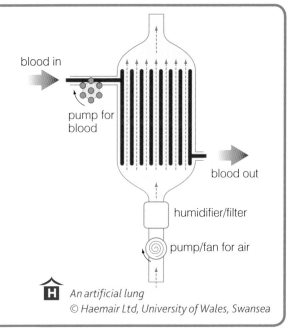

blood in

pump for blood

blood out

humidifier/filter

pump/fan for air

H *An artificial lung*
© Haemair Ltd, University of Wales, Swansea

Apply what you know

7   Look at Diagram **H** of the proposed portable lung:

a   The portable lung will be attached to the person by two tubes. Suggest the reason for this.

b   Why is filtered air pumped into the artificial lung?

c   The lung must be designed to prevent the formation of blood clots. Why is this important?

d   What will be the advantages to the patient of:

   i the portable device
   ii the internal artificial lung?

e   Suggest some obstacles the research scientists might face.

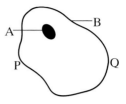

AQA Examination-style questions

Chapters 1–5

1 The cytologist is examining a sample for cancer cells.

(a) The diagram shows a normal animal cell.

Use words from the box to name structures **A** and **B**.

> cell membrane   cytoplasm   nucleus

(2 marks)

(b) Distance **P** to **Q** on the diagram is the diameter of the cell. This distance was measured on three cells using a microscope. The results were as follows:

cell 1: 63 micrometres
cell 2: 78 micrometres
cell 3: 69 micrometres

Calculate the average diameter of these cells. Show clearly how you work out your final answer.

(2 marks)

(c) The drawing on the right shows what the cytologist saw.

Give *two* differences between normal cells and the cancer cells that can be seen on the drawing.

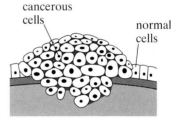

(2 marks)

(d) The drawing below shows a nerve cell:

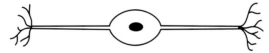

Suggest *two* ways in which this cell is specialised for transmitting information.

(2 marks)

2 Substances move in and out of our body cells.

(a) The diagram shows four ways in which molecules may move into and out of a cell.

The dots show the concentration of molecules.

The cell is respiring aerobically.

Which arrow, **A**, **B**, **C**, or **D**, represents:

(i)   movement of oxygen molecules

(ii) movement of carbon dioxide molecules?

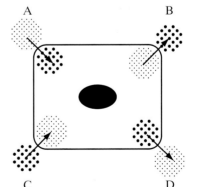

(1 mark)

(1 mark)

(b) Name the process by which these gases move into and out of the cell.

(1 mark)

(c) Patients in hospital are often given drugs dissolved in saline (sodium chloride) solution.

The graph shows the results of placing red blood cells in solutions of sodium chloride of different concentrations.

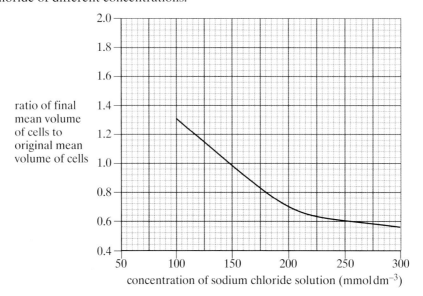

ratio of final mean volume of cells to original mean volume of cells

concentration of sodium chloride solution (mmol dm^{-3})

What concentration of sodium chloride should be used in a saline solution for use in a drip?

Explain the reasons for your answer. *(3 marks)*

3   Enzymes catalyse chemical reactions in our bodies:

(a) Egg white is a protein. Protease enzymes will digest cubes of boiled egg white.

A student investigated the effect of temperature on the digestion of egg white by protease enzyme solution.

time taken to digest egg white cubes in (minutes)

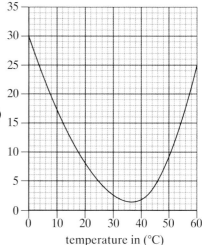

temperature in (°C)

The graph shows the student's results.

(i)   Estimate the time it would take to digest the egg white cubes at 8 °C. *(1 mark)*

(ii) At what temperature does this enzyme work best? *(1 mark)*

(iii) Why is the time taken to digest the egg white cubes greater at 60 °C than at 30 °C? *(1 mark)*

(b) In 1822, Alexis St. Martin was accidentally shot in the stomach. A doctor, called William Beaumont, looked after Alexis as the wound healed. However, the wound did not heal completely. It left a small hole through his side into his stomach. William realised that he could use the hole to study what happened to food in the human stomach.

He did many experiments with Alexis' permission. Here are two of them.

Experiment 1

William tied a piece of boiled beef to a silk thread. He then gently pushed the beef into Alexis' stomach. The piece of beef was completely digested in two hours.

Experiment 2

William removed some of Alexis' stomach juices and placed them in a test tube. The test tube was kept at 37°C. He placed a piece of raw beef in the test tube. The piece of beef was completely digested in two hours.

(i)   Why did William keep the test tube at 37°C?   *(1 mark)*

(ii) What was the dependent variable in both experiments?   *(1 mark)*

(iii) What control should William have done in Experiment 2?   *(1 mark)*

(iv) What evidence about enzymes did William's two experiments provide? *(1 mark)*

4   Our diet affects our health.

(a) Read the passage below about the diets of children in Ireland.

   A new study of teenage eating habits has revealed that one in three Irish young people do not eat any fruit, while over 50% eat too much fat.

   The teenagers were also found to be drinking, on average, one and a half glasses of soft drinks per day, but just half a glass of bottled water.

   The study revealed that since 1990, the prevalence of obesity has increased from 6% to 19% in boys and from 15% to 17% in girls.

   The study involved 450 young people, aged 13–17, from secondary schools throughout Ireland.

   A dietician is asked to prepare a leaflet for teenagers to improve their diets.

   List *five* pieces of advice about the types and quantities of food that the dietician should give in the pamphlet.   *(5 marks)*

(b) Inorganic ions form a minor but essential part of the human diet.

   Give *two* functions of each of the following ions in the human body:

   (i)   calcium   *(2 marks)*

   (ii) iron   *(2 marks)*

(c) **Table 1** shows how the estimated average daily requirements for calcium and iron in the diet vary with age and sex.

Table 1

Age (years)		Average daily requirement (mg per day)	
		calcium	iron
	1–3	275	5.3
	4–6	350	4.7
	7–10	425	6.7
Males	11–14	750	8.7
	15–18	750	8.7
	19–50	525	6.7
	50+	525	6.7
Females	11–14	625	11.4
	15–18	625	11.4
	19–50	525	11.4
	50+	525	6.7

(i)   Explain the change in the estimated average daily requirements for calcium and for iron between the ages of 4 and 10.   *(2 marks)*

(ii) Describe and explain the differences between the average daily requirements for males and females from the age of 11 for calcium and for iron.   *(4 marks)*

5   **Table 2** is from a packet of 'healthy' crisps.

Table 2

Typical nutritional values		
	Per 25 g pack	**Per 100 g**
Energy	550 kJ	2200 kJ
Protein	1.6 g	6.5 g
Carbohydrate	12.3 g	49.0 g
of which sugars	0.1 g	0.5 g
Fat	8.5 g	34.0 g
of which saturates	0.7 g	2.8 g
monounsaturates	6.8 g	27.2 g
polyunsaturates	1.0 g	4.0 g
Fibre	1.0 g	4.0 g
Sodium *	0.2 g	0.8 g
* Equivalent as salt	0.4 g	1.5 g
Guideline daily amounts		
Each day		Children
Energy		7500 kJ

(a) How much unsaturated fat is there in a 25 g packet of crisps?   *(2 marks)*

(b) How many 25 g bags of crisps would a child need to eat to get the
recommended daily amount of energy (for a child)?   *(2 marks)*

(c) The manufacturer claims that these crisps are healthier because they contain 70%
less saturated fat.

Explain why too much saturated fat is bad for us.   *(2 marks)*

(d) The manufacturer has also reduced the amount of salt in these crisps.

Why is too much salt bad for us?   *(2 marks)*

(e) The diagram shows the apparatus used to determine the energy content of samples
of food. The food is burned in oxygen and the heat released warms the water in the apparatus.

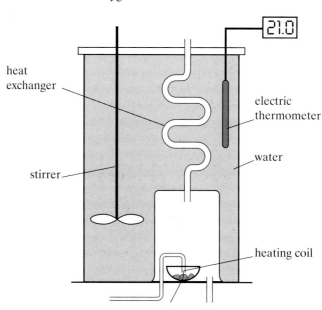

(i)   Why is the food burned in oxygen rather than in air?   *(1 mark)*

(ii)   A student investigated the energy released by burning powdered peanuts.

0.5 g of the powdered peanuts was burned in the apparatus.

The volume of water in the apparatus was 1000 cm^3.

The starting temperature of the water was 20.1 °C.

The highest temperature reached was 22.1 °C.

The energy needed to raise the temperature of 1 cm^3 water by 1 °C is 4.18 J.

1.   Calculate the amount of energy released by 100 g of peanuts. Give your answer in kilojoules and show your working.   *(2 marks)*

2.   The published value for the energy content of 100 g of peanuts is 2428 kJ.

Suggest *one* reason why the value determined in the above investigation was less than the published value.   *(1 mark)*

6   An investigation was carried out on the digestion of fat by lipase.

Milk, which contains fat, was used as the substrate.

Phenol red solution was used as an indicator.

Phenol red solution is:

yellow below pH 6.8
pink between 6.8 and 8.2
red above pH 8.2.

Sodium carbonate solution is alkaline.

Tubes **A**, **B**, **C** and **D** were set up as shown in **Table 3**.

Three drops of phenol red solution were added to each tube.

Table 3

| Tube | Volume (cm³) | | | | |
	Milk	Lipase solution	Sodium carbonate solution	Bile salts solution	Distilled water
A	5	1	1	0	2
B	5	1	1	1	1
C	5	0	1	1	2
D	5	0	1	0	3

(a)   (i)   Explain why sodium carbonate solution was added to each tube.   *(1 mark)*

(ii)   Explain why it was important that different volumes of distilled water were added to tubes **A** and **B**.   *(1 mark)*

(iii) Explain how tube **C** acted as a control.   *(1 mark)*

(b)   The tubes were kept at 35 °C for 30 minutes.

Table 4 shows the initial colour of the contents in each tube and the colour after 30 minutes.

Table 4

Tube	Initial colour	Colour after 30 minutes
A	Red	Pink
B	Red	Yellow
C	Red	Red
D	Red	Red

Explain the results for:

(i)   tube **A**   *(1 mark)*

(ii)   tube **B**   *(1 mark)*

(c) The diagram shows part of the gut wall.

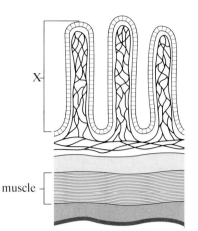

 (i) Name the structure labelled **X**. *(1 mark)*

 (ii) Describe the function of the layer of muscle. *(2 marks)*

 (iii) Describe and explain how *two* features shown in the diagram increase the rate of absorption of digested food. *(4 marks)*

 (iv) Explain how coeliac disease affects the rate of absorption of digested food. *(2 marks)*

7 Blood transports materials and helps to defend the body against infection.

The diagram shows blood as seen through a microscope:

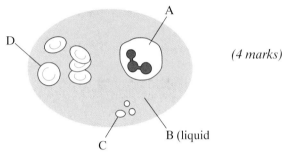

(a) Name the parts of blood **A**, **B**, **C** and **D**. *(4 marks)*

(b) When a blood sample has been collected from a patient, technicians use a haematology cell counter to count the number of each type of cell.

Table 5 shows the number of these parts in a healthy person.

Table 5

Part of blood	Number per mm³ in healthy person
White blood cells	4000 to 11 000
Red blood cells	4.5 to 6.5 million
Platelets	150 000 to 350 000

Table 6 shows the blood test results for four people.

Table 6

Test	James	John	Michael	Paul
White blood cells	6500	1000	4100	30 000
Red blood cells	5.3 million	5.2 million	3.0 million	5.5 million
Platelets	70 000	210 000	200 000	180 000

 (i) Which person is most likely to become tired quickly when exercising? *(1 mark)*

 (ii) Which person's blood is most likely to clot slowly? *(1 mark)*

 (iii) Which person is most likely to recover slowly from an infection? *(1 mark)*

(c) Plasma containing anti-A antibodies was added to blood from people of different blood groups.

The results for blood groups A and B are shown in the diagram.

The result for blood group AB has been left blank.

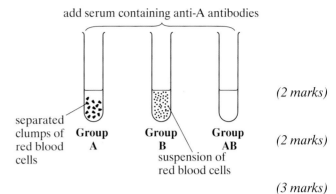

add serum containing anti-A antibodies

separated clumps of red blood cells

Group A

Group B

Group AB

suspension of red blood cells

(i) Explain why the results for blood groups A and B were different. *(2 marks)*

(ii) Describe and explain what result you would expect with the group AB blood. *(2 marks)*

(d) Explain why patients who have suffered severe burns are put on a drip containing blood plasma. *(3 marks)*

8 Heart disease caused by atheroma is becoming more common in the UK.

(a) (i) Explain the meaning of the term 'atheroma'. *(1 mark)*

(ii) Give two reasons for the increase in the incidence of atheroma. *(2 marks)*

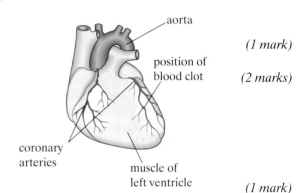

aorta

position of blood clot

coronary arteries

muscle of left ventricle

(b) The diagram shows an external view of the heart. The position of a blood clot is marked.

(i) Copy the diagram, then shade the area of the heart muscle which is likely to die as a result of the blood clot. *(1 mark)*

(ii) Explain why this area of the heart muscle is likely to die. *(1 mark)*

(c) Surgeons can take parts of veins from a patient's leg and use them to bypass a region of a coronary artery affected by atheroma.

During the operation, the heart is first connected to a heart–lung machine, and then stopped while the operation is carried out.

(i) Describe the functions of a heart–lung machine. *(3 marks)*

(ii) A miniature heart–lung machine is being developed for use in operations on children. The machine is being tested on animals. Evaluate the use of animals for testing a device such as the miniature heart–lung machine. *(5 marks)*

9 Our breathing system supplies us with oxygen and gets rid of carbon dioxide.

(a) The diagram shows part of the thorax.

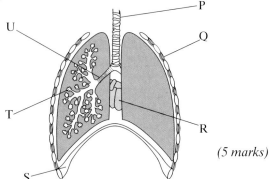

Which letter labels:

    (i)   the heart

    (ii) the trachea

    (iii) where gaseous exchange takes place

    (iv) a structure that moves upwards
         during inspiration

    (v) a structure that becomes flattened
        during inspiration?

(5 marks)

(b) Emphysema is a lung disease.

The drawings show sections through the lung of a healthy person and through the lung of a person with emphysema. The drawings are drawn to the same scale.

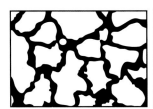
    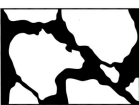

section through the lung   section through the lung
of a healthy person   of a person with emphysema

Use information from the drawings to answer the questions.

What effect does emphysema have on:

    (i)   the thickness of the surface used for gas exchange   *(1 mark)*

    (ii) the total area available for gas exchange?   *(1 mark)*

(c) A technician measured the efficiency of the lungs in two men.

The two men did the same amount of exercise.
One man was in good health. The other man had emphysema.

The results are shown in **Table 7**.

Table 7

	Man with good health	Man with emphysema
Oxygen entering blood (dm³ per minute)	2.1	1.1
Air flow into lungs (dm³ per minute)	90.7	46.0

The man in good health was able to take more oxygen into his blood than the man with emphysema.

Calculate how much more oxygen was taken into the blood per minute by the man in good health. Show your working.   *(2 marks)*

(d) The graph shows the effect of changing the concentration of carbon dioxide in inhaled air on the ventilation rate.

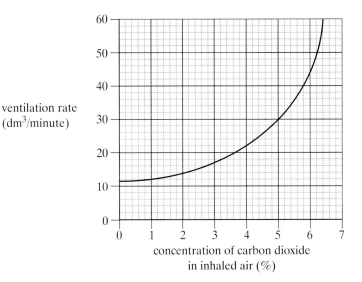

concentration of carbon dioxide
in inhaled air (%)

(i) Use the graph to calculate the percentage increase in ventilation rate when the concentration of carbon dioxide in inhaled air rises from 0 % to 5 %. Show your working. *(2 marks)*

(ii) Describe how the rise in carbon dioxide concentration of inhaled air leads to a change in the breathing rate. *(3 marks)*

(e) Read the passage below.

Paramedics are taught CPR (cardiopulmonary resuscitation), a combination of mouth-to-mouth resuscitation and chest presses.

Recently, CPR guidelines were revised to put more emphasis on chest presses. Stopping chest compressions to blow air into the lungs of someone who is unresponsive detracts from the more important task of keeping blood moving to provide oxygen and nourishment to the brain and heart.

Another big advantage to dropping the rescue breaths: It could make bystanders more willing to provide CPR in the first place.

In a new investigation, researchers in Tokyo analyzed 4068 adult patients who had cardiac arrest witnessed by bystanders. Of those, 439 received chest presses only from bystanders, and 712 received conventional CPR – presses and breaths.

Any CPR attempt improved survival odds. However, 22 percent of those who received just chest compressions survived with good neurological function compared with only 10 percent of those who received combination CPR.

They concluded 'Eliminating the need for mouth-to-mouth ventilation will dramatically increase the occurrence of bystander-initiated resuscitation efforts and will increase survival.'

Use information from the passage to evaluate the recent change to CPR guidelines for paramedics. *(4 marks)*

6.1 Excretion

Cells produce a range of waste materials, **excretory products**, which must be removed from the body. Toxic (poisonous) substances, e.g. alcohol, must also be removed or cells become damaged. The table shows the main excretory products and the organs which remove them.

Excretory product	Excretory organ	Excreted in
carbon dioxide	lungs	exhaled air
urea	kidney	urine
mineral salts	skin and kidney	sweat and urine
water	skin, kidney, lungs	sweat, urine, exhaled air

Urea is produced in the **liver** from the breakdown of surplus amino acids (see Diagram **A**). It is carried to the **kidneys** where it is filtered from the blood. We have two kidneys which produce **urine** and pass it to the bladder for storage. The kidneys contain millions of microscopic filters which allow dissolved materials to pass through them under pressure. Protein molecules and blood cells are too large to pass through the filter (see Diagram **B**).

Useful substances, such as sugar and dissolved ions, are also filtered and must be reabsorbed back into the blood. Most of the filtered water is also reabsorbed. Urine contains urea, the remaining salts and water and other chemicals, including those made from alcohol and drugs.

Objectives

What are the excretory organs?

Where is urea made?

How do the kidneys work?

How do the kidneys maintain homeostasis?

What is dialysis?

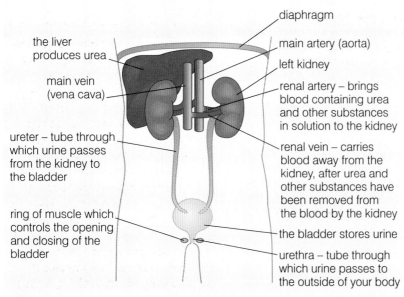

the liver produces urea

main vein (vena cava)

ureter – tube through which urine passes from the kidney to the bladder

ring of muscle which controls the opening and closing of the bladder

diaphragm

main artery (aorta)

left kidney

renal artery – brings blood containing urea and other substances in solution to the kidney

renal vein – carries blood away from the kidney, after urea and other substances have been removed from the blood by the kidney

the bladder stores urine

urethra – tube through which urine passes to the outside of your body

 A *The excretory system*

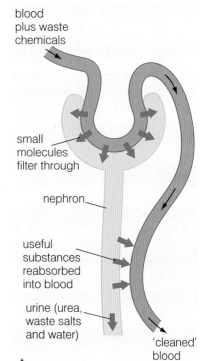

blood plus waste chemicals

small molecules filter through

nephron

useful substances reabsorbed into blood

urine (urea, waste salts and water)

'cleaned' blood

B *A single kidney nephron*

Sitting higher tier

Water balance

The water and solute balance in the body needs to be kept fairly constant for cells to stay healthy. When we breathe out, water is lost to the air and we also sweat more when we are hot, losing water from the skin (see page 59, Diagram **B**). Water is also lost in faeces. The kidneys are able to balance the water and mineral content of the blood. When we are short of water, due to increased sweating, the kidneys reabsorb more and we produce less urine. This is an example of homeostasis (see page 58).

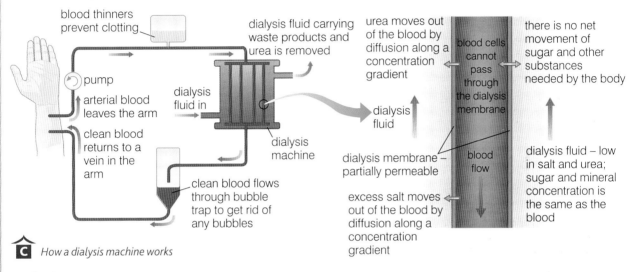

C *How a dialysis machine works*

Dialysis

When kidneys fail to work, urea and other toxins, plus large amounts of water, build up in the blood and this can prove fatal.

Dialysis machines which mimic the role of the kidneys (referred to as **haemodialysis**) are used to treat kidney failure.

In the machine, the blood and dialysis fluid are separated by partially permeable membranes. Urea and other wastes substances diffuse from the blood to the fluid. Useful substances remain in the blood by controlling their concentration in the dialysis fluid. Excess water leaves the blood by osmosis and the patient may lose weight during dialysis as a consequence.

The main disadvantage of the machine is that the patient must be connected for 4 to 5 hours, often in a hospital, three times a week.

Another common treatment is **peritoneal dialysis**, which can be done in the patient's home in the body. In the abdomen the peritoneal membrane lies around the intestines and is used as the partially permeable membrane. Dialysis fluid is inserted into the abdominal cavity, waste materials diffuse out of the blood, through the peritoneal membrane into the cavity. Then the fluid plus waste is drained away.

Many health problems result when toxic materials, including alcohol, accumulate in the blood and interfere with the cell processes. Laboratory technicians detect toxins such as alcohol and drugs in blood, urine, breath and saliva and supply data to doctors and forensic scientists. Where kidneys have been damaged by toxins or infection, doctors use dialysis or kidney transplantation to ensure that urea and other waste materials can be removed from the patient's blood. Scientists are involved in designing and maintaining dialysis and operating equipment.

Scientists@work

Some patients are considered suitable for a kidney **transplant** but they may have to wait for a **donor**.

The table shows advantages and disadvantages of types of treatment for kidney disease.

Type of treatment	Advantages	Disadvantages
Kidney transplant	**Recipient** freed from dependency on machines Long term costs less than dialysis: £5000 per year for drugs Diet less restricted	Risk of rejection so need immunosuppressant drugs Costs about £17 000 per patient Check-ups needed Availability of donors
Haemodialysis	Patient kept alive while waiting for transplant Suitable for patients with abdominal scars and wounds who cannot have peritoneal dialysis	Many visits to hospital Restricts holidays to places with kidney machine Costs £35 000 per year Possible infection from equipment Availability of machines and expert staff Some dietary restrictions
Peritoneal dialysis	Patient kept alive while waiting for transplant Can be done at home at times to suit, by the patient Only bags of fluid needed when travelling Diet may be less restricted than when on haemodialysis	Patient must maintain strict hygienic conditions Costs £17 500 per year Not suitable for people with abdominal wounds or scars Regular monitoring

AQA Examiner's tip

- Urea is made in the liver.
- Protein is too big to be filtered.
- Useful glucose is filtered by the kidney and must be reabsorbed.
- **Excretion** is removal of waste made by cells.
- Urine is a solution containing urea.

There is a direct relationship between blood alcohol concentration and ability to drive safely. Alcohol levels in the body can be measured in blood, urine, breath or saliva. To produce reliable data, scientists have performed thousands of tests for comparison. They have shown that accurate breath tests are a good indicator of blood alcohol concentration. Urine tests indicate the presence of alcohol but are not equivalent to blood concentrations. Saliva tests involve an enzyme reaction on a testing strip and can be affected by temperature, making them unreliable.

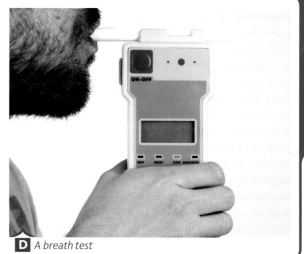

D A breath test

How science works

Practical activity

Do not forget to make careful observations and recordings

During your practical work you may be asked to use food tests to identify artificial blood, filtrate and urine. Remember that blood contains protein and glucose, filtrate will not contain protein because the molecules are too big to be filtered and urine will not contain glucose because it has been reabsorbed. This could be a PSA or an ISA.

Apply what you know

1 How will your kidneys respond:
a if you drink a lot on a cold day?
b if you exercise vigorously?

2 During dialysis, by what process does:
a urea, and   b water,   leave the blood?

3 Urine tests are not accurate indicators of how much alcohol is in a person's blood. Why will levels of alcohol in the urine be different from that in the blood?

4 Evaluate the benefits of a kidney transplant rather than dialysis for a patient with kidney disease.

5 Currently there are over 6000 people waiting for a kidney transplant. What is the annual cost, if 80% are on haemodialysis and 20% on peritoneal dialysis? What would be the annual drug cost if all 6000 had a transplant? How could the UK government increase the number of donors? Can you think of any ethical issues concerned with transplants?

7 The nervous system, hormones and coordination

7.1 The nervous system

Health professionals need to understand how the body detects and responds to changing conditions, both internal and external.

The nervous system and hormones enable the body to respond to external changes and to control the environment inside the body. For example, it is very important that your cells are kept warm enough for enzymes to work, so you have sensory cells in the skin to detect temperature changes. Other sensory cells are found in the eye, ear, nose and tongue to detect light, sound and chemicals.

Objectives

How does the body detect stimuli?

How does the body respond to stimuli?

What are reflex and voluntary actions?

The nervous system

The brain, spinal cord and nerves form the nervous system. The **brain** is vital for coordinating many actions and for thinking and learning. Together, the brain and spinal cord form the **central nervous system (CNS)** which receives electrical impulses from **sensory nerves** and sends electrical impulses to all parts of the body via the **motor nerves**. **Nerves** are bundles of **neurones** (nerve cells). Both reflex and voluntary actions involve sensory and motor neurones which may be linked by **relay** neurones.

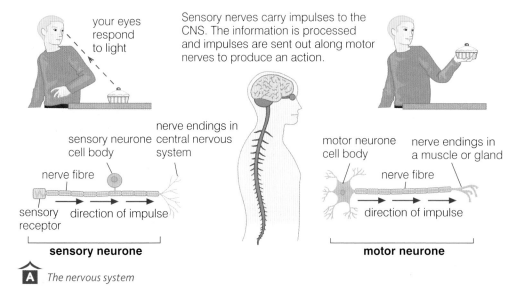

Sensory nerves carry impulses to the CNS. The information is processed and impulses are sent out along motor nerves to produce an action.

your eyes respond to light

nerve endings in central nervous system

sensory neurone cell body

nerve fibre

sensory receptor

direction of impulse

sensory neurone

motor neurone cell body

nerve endings in a muscle or gland

nerve fibre

direction of impulse

motor neurone

A The nervous system

Voluntary actions start when your brain thinks about what you want to do, e.g. if you see some litter on the floor you may decide to pick it up or leave it.

Other reactions happen automatically and often help to protect the body from danger. These are called **reflex actions** and are rapid responses to external stimuli, e.g. if you touch something hot your hand will be moved away rapidly by the pulling action of the arm muscles.

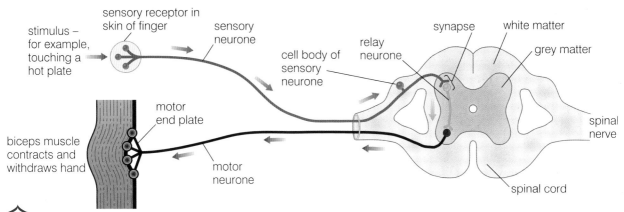

B *A reflex action*

Receptors at the beginning of **sensory** neurones in the skin may detect heat or other external stimuli, e.g. touch. But you also have receptors inside the body to detect changes in pH when carbon dioxide levels go up, for example, or to detect pressure changes in the blood vessels.

The muscles are **effectors** because they cause the arm to move. Some glands in the body may also act as effectors. The **synapses** are tiny gaps between the neurones where the electrical impulse stimulates the production of a chemical which crosses the gap.

Apply what you know

Nervous actions can be summed up by the following sequence:

stimulus → receptor → coordination → effector → response
system

The table shows some examples:

Stimulus	Receptor	Coordination system	Effector	Response
Hot plate	Temperature receptors in skin	Relay neurone in CNS (spinal cord)	Biceps muscle	Arm pulled
Bright light	Light receptors in retina of eye	Relay neurone in CNS (non-thinking part of brain)	Muscles of iris	Pupil is made smaller
Cake on a plate	Light receptors in retina of eye	Brain	Muscles in arm	Pick up cake
Crumb of cake	In trachea	Relay neurone	Muscles of rib cage	Cough

1 For each example, state if it is a voluntary or reflex action.

2 How does each of the reflex actions protect the body?

PSA or ISA

You will have the opportunity to investigate some stimuli.

Touch

You can determine which parts of the skin contain the most touch receptors by using callipers which have two pointed tips. Fix the calliper points 10 mm apart. Touch the back of the hand of a blindfolded subject. The subject tells you if they can feel one or two points. If 'one', then widen the callipers and try again; repeat until the answer is 'two' and record the distance. If the answer is 'two', then narrow the callipers and test again. Try on different areas of the hand. The most sensitive area is where 2 points can be detected with the smallest tip separation; this is likely to be 2–3 mm.

Light

Sit a subject facing away from a window for at least two minutes. Hold a ruler in front of their eyes and estimate the width of the pupils. Shine a torch in one eye. Record what happens to the pupil. Do both pupils change equally? How long does it take for the pupil to return to its original width?

Try to relate the experiments to your knowledge of the nervous system.

The brain coordinates information from many parts of the body, including the eye, ear, tongue, nose and skin. These **sense organs** are designed to ensure that external stimuli such as light, sound, chemicals, touch and temperature are directed to receptor cells and detected. The **eye** is designed to focus light onto the receptor cells in the retina.

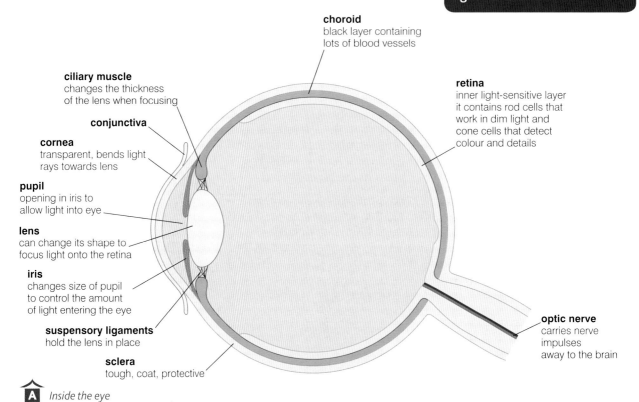

choroid
black layer containing lots of blood vessels

ciliary muscle
changes the thickness of the lens when focusing

conjunctiva

cornea
transparent, bends light rays towards lens

pupil
opening in iris to allow light into eye

lens
can change its shape to focus light onto the retina

iris
changes size of pupil to control the amount of light entering the eye

suspensory ligaments
hold the lens in place

sclera
tough, coat, protective

retina
inner light-sensitive layer it contains rod cells that work in dim light and cone cells that detect colour and details

optic nerve
carries nerve impulses away to the brain

A *Inside the eye*

Normally the light rays from an object are bent and focused on the **retina** by the **cornea** and **lens**, to form an image.

The cornea cannot change shape so the lens has to be altered to focus on distant or near objects. To look at a distant object the lens is relatively thin but when you read a book the **ciliary muscles** contract, which causes the **suspensory ligaments** to slacken, and the lens becomes fatter.

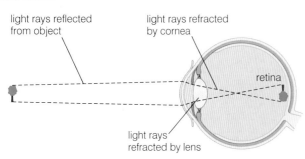

light rays reflected from object

light rays refracted by cornea

retina

light rays refracted by lens

B *Focussing*

Find out ...

Safety at work

Good lighting, particularly natural light, helps to reduce accidents and increase productivity in the workplace. Blue-enriched light appears to improve alertness and mood! But too much light can damage eyes. Workers in noisy factories often wear ear protectors. Find out how other workers protect their sense organs from external stimuli.

Sitting higher tier

When optometrists find out that you cannot focus properly, they will prescribe correcting lenses. Short sight occurs when the eyeball is too long and the light rays focus in front of the retina. Long sight is usually caused by a short eyeball or flatness of the cornea. The rays come to a focus behind the retina. The optometrist will prescribe spectacle or contact lenses to correct these conditions.

short sight

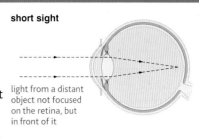

light from a distant object not focused on the retina, but in front of it

concave (diverging) correcting lens

light from a distant object now focused on the retina

Scientists@work

Optometrists perform eye tests to check that you can focus properly, but they are also trained to detect changes in the eye which may be from a variety of causes.

A **cataract** occurs when the lens becomes cloudy due to a build-up of protein. Ophthalmic surgeons can replace cloudy lenses with a clear plastic one in around 15 minutes. When corneas have age-related damage, the light cannot pass through to the retina. Healthy tissue from a donor is needed to replace a layer of cells which line the inside of the cornea. Many organ donors also donate their corneas.

Damage to the small blood vessels in the retina (called retinopathy) can be the result of high blood sugar in someone with diabetes or high blood pressure. Optometrists test eye pressures by puffing air into the eye to help diagnose these conditions.

Sometimes the optometrist can diagnose an illness before other, more severe symptoms, arise. Dr Lee Goldstein, an American psychiatrist, discovered that early Alzheimer's disease can be detected in the eyes by identifying a particular protein which is normally found in the brain of these patients. Alzheimer's disease is a form of dementia involving severe memory loss. Patients often become completely dependent on others for their everyday needs. If diagnosed early, drugs are available to slow the progression of this distressing disease.

long sight

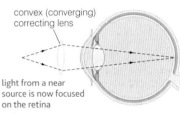

light from a near source is not focused on the retina but behind the retina

convex (converging) correcting lens

light from a near source is now focused on the retina

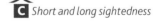

C *Short and long sightedness*

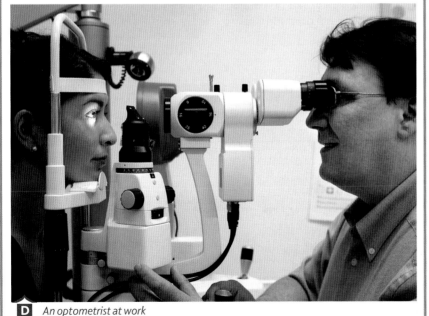

D *An optometrist at work*

AQA Examiner's tip

- Always relate the function to the structure of parts of the eye.
- Learn which lenses are used to correct long and short sight.

Find out ...

What are the benefits of cataract operations and corneal transplants?

Apply what you know

1 What changes in the eye could result in blindness?

Many of your body processes are controlled by chemicals called **hormones**. Hormones are produced by **endocrine glands**.

When an endocrine gland is stimulated by chemical changes in the blood, or by nerve impulses, it releases its hormone directly into the bloodstream. The hormone is carried by the **blood** to a **target organ**. The target organ will then respond.

Sometimes the whole body is affected by a particular hormone. The pituitary gland releases growth hormone which stimulates growth of the whole body, particularly of bones, in childhood. Growth hormone has many other function in adults, which include increasing the mass of muscles.

Other hormones target specific organs, e.g. glucagon, produced by the pancreas, targets the liver; follicle stimulating hormone (FSH) from the pituitary gland targets the ovary or testis.

The effect of hormones can be short term or long term. When adrenaline is released during a time of stress it causes an increase in heart rate, breathing rate, blood sugar and blood pressure. The effect of adrenaline usually lasts for just a few minutes, but the effect of growth hormone on increasing bone length will be permanent.

Too much or too little hormone can cause medical problems for the person, e.g. if the pancreas produces too little insulin the blood sugar levels rise to a dangerous level resulting in diabetes; too much growth hormone may cause a person to become a giant. **Endocrinologists** are doctors who investigate imbalances in hormones, which can be very complex, but most doctors have many diabetic patients on their lists and know how to treat this common condition.

Objectives

What are hormones?

What do hormones do?

How is blood sugar controlled?

What is negative feedback?

AQA Examiner's tip

- Learn to label a diagram of the endocrine glands.
- Make sure you know one function for each gland.

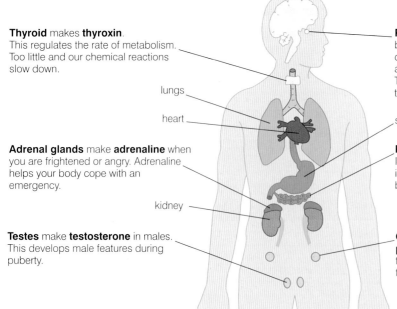

Thyroid makes **thyroxin**. This regulates the rate of metabolism. Too little and our chemical reactions slow down.

lungs

heart

Adrenal glands make **adrenaline** when you are frightened or angry. Adrenaline helps your body cope with an emergency.

kidney

Testes make **testosterone** in males. This develops male features during puberty.

Pituitary is a gland at the base of the brain. It makes many hormones and controls things like growth, water balance and sperm and egg production. The pituitary also makes hormones that control other endocrine glands.

stomach

Pancreas makes **insulin** and **glucagon**. Insulin lowers blood sugar by changing it to glycogen. Glucagon increases blood sugar.

Ovaries make **oestrogen** and **progesterone** in females. These control the menstrual cycle and develop female features during puberty.

A *Endocrine system*

B *The main endocrine organs, some hormones they produce and their functions*

Gland	Hormone(s)	Target organ(s)	Effect of hormone
Pituitary	Many hormones	Other endocrine glands	Causes glands to secrete their hormone
Pituitary	Growth hormone	Whole body	Stimulates growth
Pituitary	FSH and LH	Ovary	Involved in controlling menstrual cycle (see page 76)
Thyroid	Thyroxin	All body cells	Controls metabolic rate
Pancreas	Insulin	All body cells	Cells absorb glucose and convert it to glycogen
Pancreas	Glucagon	Liver	Liver changes glycogen to glucose
Adrenal glands	Adrenaline	Liver, heart, lungs	Increases blood sugar, heart rate and breathing rate
Ovaries	Oestrogen and progesterone	Whole body	Controls female sexual development
Testes	Testosterone	Whole body	Controls male sexual characteristics

Did you know ???????

Insulin causes fat and muscle cells to absorb blood sugar. The fat cells convert sugar to fat for storage. The muscle cells have a ready supply of energy for contraction.

Did you know ???????

The four common symptoms of diabetes are:

- being thirsty a lot of the time
- passing large amounts of urine
- tiredness
- weight loss.

Diabetes

There are two types of diabetes. In Type 1, the pancreas stops producing insulin. This usually occurs in young people and develops very quickly. Type 1 is treated with insulin injections and a healthy diet.

Type 2 diabetes develops gradually and either the pancreas does not produce enough insulin or the liver and other cells become 'insulin resistant' and do not absorb the blood sugar. Weight control, diet and physical activity are the first treatments, but if these do not reduce the blood sugar sufficiently the patient may need medication.

Insulin can be given in several ways, but not in tablet form because the hormone is made of protein and would be digested. Injections can be delivered by syringes, pens and pumps; there are forms of insulin which can be inhaled and microjets linked to 'watches' which pulse insulin into the skin at timed intervals. These days insulin is produced by genetic engineering (see page 82). For the future it is hoped stem cell therapy will offer a cure for diabetes.

Banting and Best

Banting and **Best** were awarded the Nobel prize for their work on extracting insulin. Banting had realised that digestive juices in the pancreas destroyed the hormone when other scientists tried to extract it from a complete pancreas. They decided to tie off the pancreatic duct in healthy dogs. This meant the cells producing digestive juice withered away. The cells which were left, called islet cells, were removed, mashed up and the extract was injected into diabetic dogs. The dogs recovered. More than 15 million people living today would have died if insulin had not been discovered.

Scientists@work

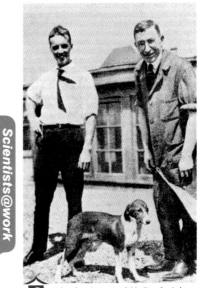

C   *Charles Best and Sir Frederick Banting*

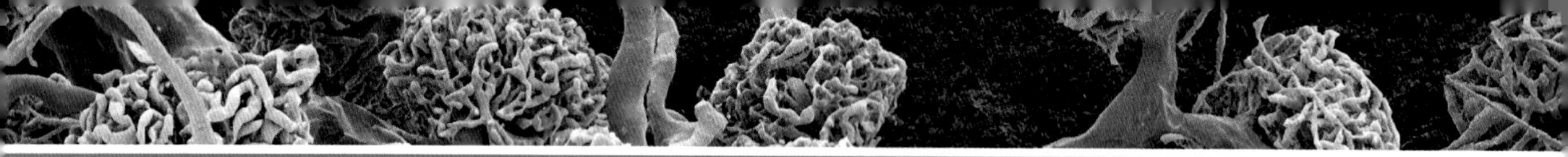

1. Make a list of the ways in which control by the endocrine system is different from the nervous system. Think about speed, what is targeted and how long the effect lasts.

2. Decide which of the following are controlled by the nervous system and which by the endocrine system:
   - blinking,
   - blood sugar concentration,
   - flinching from a loud noise,
   - growing,
   - menstrual cycle,
   - sneezing when inhaling pepper,
   - focusing on a book to read it,
   - swatting a fly,
   - metabolic rate.

3. Banting and Best used dogs in their experiments. At one time insulin was extracted from pig pancreas to treat humans. Nowadays human insulin is made using genetically engineered bacteria. Evaluate the pros and cons of these procedures.

   When you evaluate this information remember to give a balanced argument.

   What were the benefits of using animals? What reasons would some people give for objecting? Why is human insulin better than pig insulin? Think of the quantities of insulin which are needed.

Sitting higher tier

Blood sugar control

Insulin and glucagon are produced by patches of cells in the pancreas called **islets**. Beta cells in the islets have receptors to detect high concentrations of glucose, the stimulus. Insulin is released in response to this stimulus. Receptors on the surface of the liver cells (and also muscle and fat cells) combine with the insulin and this triggers the cells to absorb the glucose. The fall in glucose concentration means the beta cells are no longer stimulated and stop producing insulin. Low glucose concentrations are detected by receptors on alpha cells in the islets resulting in glucagon secretion. Glucagon causes the liver to change glycogen to glucose. Consequently the blood glucose concentration rises again.

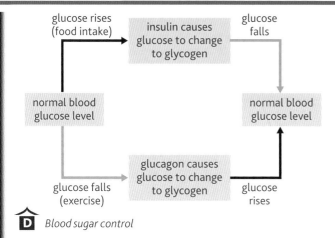

D *Blood sugar control*

Negative feedback

Blood sugar falls after insulin is released – this removes the stimulus so the beta cells stop releasing insulin. This is an example of negative feedback.

The pituitary gland releases **antidiuretic hormone (ADH)** when receptors in part of the brain, the **hypothalamus**, detect that the water content of the blood is too low. ADH travels to the kidneys and causes them to reabsorb more water, reducing the volume of the urine. The stimulus (low water) is removed so the pituitary stops producing ADH.

> **Hint**
>
> Remember: an increase in blood sugar causes a release of insulin. The insulin reduces blood sugar which stops the release of more insulin. This is negative feedback.

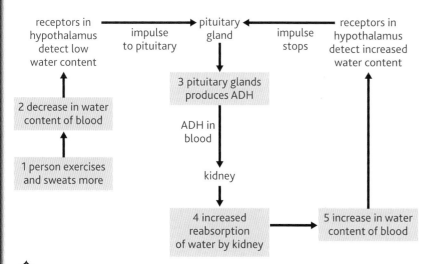

E   *This is the way the body controls water concentration in the blood. It is an example of negative feedback*

Apply what you know

4   What are the advantages of the changes caused by adrenaline to someone who is frightened by a wild animal and wants to run away? Relate your answer to the extra energy required.

5   Look at Diagram **E**. What would happen if at point 1 the person sat down and drank 1 litre of water?

6   There may be a delay of about 20 minutes before the kidney responds to a person drinking more water. Can you suggest why?

7.4　Homeostasis

In the previous chapters you will have seen how various conditions are controlled inside the body. The way the body maintains a constant internal environment is referred to as **homeostasis**.

Cell reactions are affected by changes in factors such as temperature, pH and water content. The purpose of homeostasis is to keep these within narrow limits. Other examples of things which need to be kept constant are blood sugar, ion and carbon dioxide concentrations.

The blood has a very important role in homeostasis because it carries materials and heat. Heat produced in the liver and muscles will raise the core temperature and reach all parts of the body in the blood.

Body temperature

If your body temperature rises above 37°C the warmer blood flows to the brain. **Receptors** in the **thermoregulatory** centre of the brain are sensitive to blood temperature so they detect the increase. The brain responds by sending nerve impulses to the body organs which need to act to bring the temperature back to normal.

When you get hot your skin looks very red and you sweat more. Sweating helps to cool the body because the water in sweat evaporates, using heat from the skin to do so.

When you sweat you lose a lot of water, so the kidneys produce less urine to reduce water loss from excretion. The brain will detect that you need water so you feel thirsty and drink.

The thermoregulatory centre also receives impulses from temperature receptors in the **skin**. This means the brain has information about the body's core and surface temperature.

Marathon runners rely on data from sports scientists to help them train for races. There are many variables to consider, including training methods and sports equipment. But however well-trained an athlete may be he, or she, must understand the importance of homeostasis.

If the core body temperature rises by one or two degrees, the athlete will sweat profusely and is in danger of dehydration which leads to heat exhaustion. Scientists have worked out the optimum water intake before and during races to reduce this risk, particularly on a hot day. Food scientists have produced sports drinks which contain sugar and ions. These are useful, alongside pure water, in long races to supply energy, maintain the water-solute balance in the blood, and reduce the risk of dehydration.

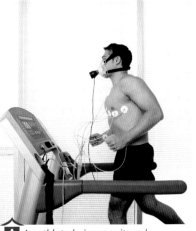
A *An athlete being monitored*

Sitting higher tier

In 7.3 you learnt that the hypothalamus detects the water content of the blood. **Osmoregulation** is a good example of how negative feedback ensures homeostasis.

The **hypothalamus** also contains the thermoregulatory centre with temperature receptors. When the blood temperature rises, impulses pass from the brain to arterioles in the skin. These dilate which increases the blood flow to the skin capillaries giving the skin a red appearance. Heat from the blood is lost from the skin by radiation. The sweat glands are stimulated by the nervous system to release more sweat leading to a reduction in core temperature.

When you are too cold the arterioles constrict, sweating reduces and impulses from the brain cause your muscles to 'shiver', releasing heat energy from the contracting muscles.

Did you know

Heat receptors are concentrated in the fingertips, nose, and elbows. Cold receptors are concentrated in the upper lip, nose, chin, chest and fingers.

Foul facts

In the heat wave of August 2003, about 13 000 people in France died of hyperthermia (overheating).

Scientists@work

About 1 in 4 people, mostly young adults, suffer shivering following an operation. This can be due to a drop in core body temperature during the operation. Nurses keep the patient warm with blankets and warm fluids and usually give extra oxygen via a mask.

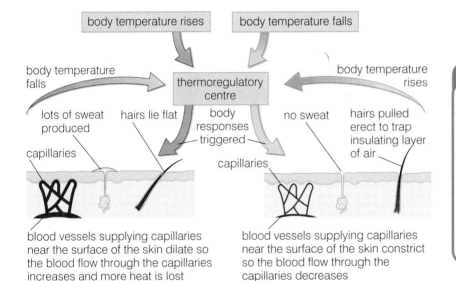

B *How body temperature is controlled*

Apply what you know

1. What happens to cells if the fluid around them has a high concentration of sugar or ions?

2. Why do you pass more urine during the winter time?

3. Suggest why the soles of your feet are less sensitive to external heat than your fingertips.

4. Why is it more difficult to lose the heat from your skin when you wear clothes?

5. Why do marathon runners drink water during a race?

6. Why is it important to keep the patient warm after an operation?

7. Why does the patient need extra oxygen after an operation?

8. When walkers are caught out by sudden bad weather the survival advice is to stay put and shelter rather than risk a long walk in the cold. More people have died from hypothermia by trying to keep going. Can you explain why keeping going increases the risk of hypothermia?

8 Muscles, bones and movement

8.1 Bones, muscles and joints

Back pain is the major cause of absence from work. Most injuries suffered by humans involve the **bones**, **joints** and **muscles**. To understand how these occur you need to learn some basic facts about these structures.

Bones

The **human skeleton** has several important functions:

- It gives **shape** to the body.
- It gives **support** by allowing us to stand upright.
- It supports and **protects** softer organs.
- It acts as an attachment point for muscles, which enable us to **move.**
- The bone marrow inside long bones **produces red and white blood cells**.

Bones contain living cells which make hard bone by incorporating minerals such as calcium salts. New bone can be made when old bone is reabsorbed or bone is damaged. We have over 200 bones in our body.

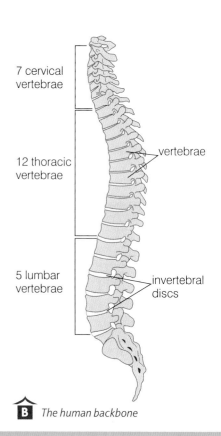

skull
jaw bone
collar bone
shoulder blade
breast bone
humerus
rib cage
back bone
radius
hip (pelvis)
ulna
hand bones
femur
knee cap
fibula
tibia

7 cervical vertebrae

12 thoracic vertebrae

vertebrae

5 lumbar vertebrae

invertebral discs

A *The human skeleton*

B *The human backbone*

Joints

We are able to move about because we have joints and muscles to pull the bones. Diagram **C** shows a **synovial joint** which is designed to move easily. The knee is the largest synovial joint; others are the shoulder and finger joints.

- **Ligaments** are strong bands of connective tissue which hold bones together; they are slightly elastic to allow movement.
- **Cartilage** covers the ends of bones; it is smooth to reduce friction and acts as a shock absorber.
- **Synovial fluid** also reduces friction by lubricating the joint.

Other joints may have little movement (vertebrae) or no movement (between skull bones). **Discs of cartilage** cushion the vertebrae and act as shock absorbers when you jump about.

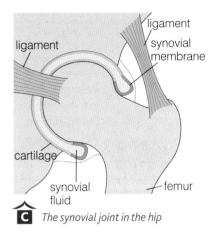

C *The synovial joint in the hip*

Muscles

Muscles are attached to bones by very tough **tendons**. Your muscles are arranged in **antagonistic** pairs. When one of these muscles (the flexor) contracts a bending action will occur. To straighten the limb again the other muscle (the extensor) must contract to pull the bones back. Try to work out which muscles are pulling to bend and straighten your leg or your fingers. Diagram **D** shows the action of the arm muscles which pull across the elbow joint to move your lower arm up and down.

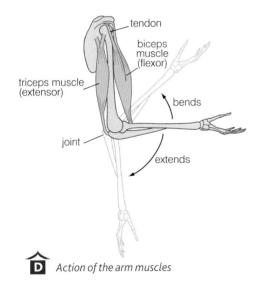

D *Action of the arm muscles*

When a muscle is not contracting it is relaxed, but most muscles have cells which are contracted to maintain the **posture** of the body. Muscle tone is the amount of tension in your muscles and you would be very floppy without it. Your head is supported by the tension in the neck muscles, so if you fall asleep in a chair your head flops forwards.

8.2 Skeletal health

Good posture means that your bones are in the correct position and consequently so are your internal organs. The vertebral column should have three natural curves and the line between the shoulders should be level. Poor posture can lead to back pain; lifting and bending incorrectly can also result in back injuries.

Some people suffer a 'slipped' or prolapsed disc when they lift things or turn awkwardly. The cartilage bulges out and may press on a nerve causing pain. This can be seen in Diagram **B**.

Scientists@work

Physiotherapists assess and treat people whose movement is restricted. They use exercise, massage, hydrotherapy, deep heat and ultrasound to treat injuries or disorders of muscles and joints.

Chiropractors and **osteopaths** use their hands to manipulate joints and muscles to treat backache, neck pains and other injuries. The chiropractor works mainly on the vertebral column, but also assesses the whole body to make sure the bones are in the correct position. The osteopath also has this holistic (whole body) approach and may use deep massage to encourage full movement and improve the function of the muscles, ligaments and bones.

Physiotherapists, chiropractors and osteopaths may use different methods, but all attempt to return the muscles and skeleton to their correct position after injury.

Injuries to parts of joints

Sprains are damage to ligaments – usually due to overstretching and tearing the ligament fibres. Sometimes the bones may **dislocate** (move out of place) if the ligament is sprained. These are common injuries in sport.

Fractures are damage to bones. These can occur due to an accident or may be due to a degenerative condition of the bone called **osteoporosis**. This occurs when you make too little bone, lose too much bone or both. It is important to have sufficient calcium in the diet to make the bone hard and strong.

Strains are damage to muscle from stretching and tearing.

Tendons can be inflamed due to overuse or ill-fitting trainers, as in Achilles tendonitis at the back of the heel.

Cartilage can be damaged suddenly or by gradual wear and tear. This can cause pain and difficulty in moving the joint and may lead to a condition called **osteoarthritis**.

Find out ...

Safety in the workplace

Who is responsible for back injuries that occur at work? Discuss the role of employers and personal responsibility for safety when putting stress on the spine at work. Look at the two examples:

- Nurses use hoists to lift patients who cannot walk.
- Chairs should be designed to give maximum support when sitting at a computer.

Objectives

Why is good posture important?

How are muscles, bones and joints damaged by disease and injury?

The wrong way!

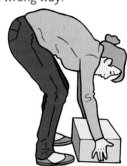

The right way!

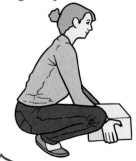

 How to avoid injury when bending and lifting

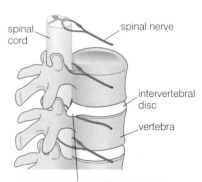

spinal cord

spinal nerve

intervertebral disc

vertebra

part of the softer middle disc bulges through the fibrous outer ring and presses on the nerve as it leaves the spinal cord

B *Prolapsed inter-vertebral disc*

Orthopaedic surgeons repair damaged joints using **keyhole surgery.** This aids a speedy recovery as only small incisions are made, reducing damage to the surrounding tissues. Sometimes a joint replacement is necessary – usually of the hip or knee. Metal covered by plastic is traditionally used to construct the head of the bone. The materials in the joint must not cause the body to react against them and must mimic the natural joint. The metal replaces bone and gives strength to the joint, while the plastic cover replaces cartilage to reduce friction between the parts.

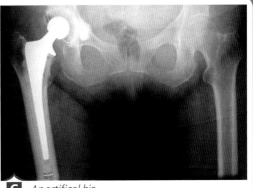

C   *An artifical hip*

Practical activity

Analysing bone structure

When a piece of bone is burned the organic compounds, which contain carbon, are removed. The remaining ash contains minerals including calcium salts.

When bone is placed in acid the mineral salts dissolve and leave behind the organic compounds such as protein. The shape of the bone is kept, but it becomes flexible and easily bent.

If you try this experiment, remember the safety rules and make careful observations and recordings. This could be a PSA.

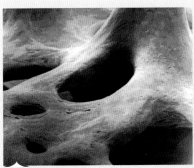

D   *Normal bone*

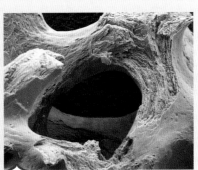

E   *Osteoporotic bone*

Apply what you know

1   Why will osteoarthritis make moving difficult and painful?

2   What would happen if you placed the ash from burned bone into acid?

3   A woman visited her doctor complaining of backache and pain in her knee joints. The doctor suggested she should increase foods containing calcium in her diet and lose some weight, stop carrying her heavy shoulder bag and do more light exercise. He also recommended she visit a physiotherapist. Suggest reasons for this advice.

4   Osteoporosis is a degenerative bone condition. Look at Photos **D** and **E** of normal and osteoporotic bone.

a   Give two visible differences in the bone.

b   Suggest why people with osteoporosis suffer from broken bones.

Did you know ??????

Every year about 5 million working days are lost in the UK due to back pain and it costs the NHS more than £1 billion to treat back-related problems.

Foul facts

Smoking slows down the activity of bone-building cells, which increases your risk of broken bones.

Hint

Always relate features of an artificial joint to the synovial joint.

Think about strength and reduced friction.

Did you know ??????

All animals with skeletons are prone to osteoarthritis – with the exception of bats and sloths, and that's because they spend so much time hanging upside-down!

Chapters 6–8

1   The diagram shows the amount of water lost by an adult in one day.

The width of the arrows shows how much water is lost in each way.

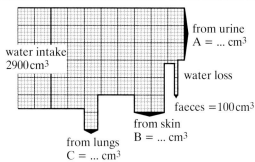

from urine
A = ... cm³

water intake
2900 cm³

water loss

faeces = 100 cm³

from skin
B = ... cm³

from lungs
C = ... cm³

(a) Calculate, from the diagram, the water loss for urine, skin and lungs.   (4 marks)

(b) When it is hot, much more water is lost from the skin. Which other method of water loss would also change significantly?

Explain your answer.   (3 marks)

(c) (i) Urine is made in the kidneys and stored for a few hours before being released from the body. In which of the following organs of the body is urine stored?

bladder   large intestine   liver   (1 mark)

(ii) Which *two* of the following substances are *not* found in the urine of a healthy person?

glucose   mineral ions   protein   urea   (2 marks)

(d) A person with kidney disease may be treated by dialysis or by having a kidney transplant.

Read the following information about dialysis and kidney transplants.

A person needs 3 dialysis sessions a week, each lasting about 8 hours.

Intake of protein and salt in the food is kept low between dialysis sessions.

For each patient, haemodialysis costs around £30 000 per year.

The use of a general anaesthetic can sometimes cause brain damage.

Drugs to suppress the immune system are given after a kidney transplant.

A transplant costs £20 000 in the first year plus £6500 in each of the following years for drugs.

Use this information to answer the questions.

(i) Give *two* advantages of treatment by having a kidney transplant rather than treatment by dialysis.   (2 marks)

(ii) Give *one* disadvantage of treatment by having a kidney transplant.   (1 mark)

(e) **Table 1** shows the amounts of some substances in the blood of one patient before dialysis and after dialysis.

Table 1

Substance	Concentration in blood plasma (g/dm³)	
	Before dialysis	**After dialysis**
Sodium ions	2.88	3.00
Potassium ions	0.22	0.14
Urea	4.50	0.30

During dialysis, substances are removed from the blood.

   (i)   Which substance in the table decreased in concentration the most during dialysis? *(1 mark)*

  (ii)   By how much did the concentration of this substance decrease? *(1 mark)*

2   Drinking alcohol regularly damages health.

  (a)   The graph shows changes in death rate from chronic liver disease between 1970 and 2000.

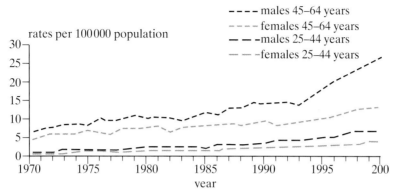

- - - - males 45–64 years
- - - - females 45–64 years
— — -males 25–44 years
— — -females 25–44 years

   (i)   In a city of 2 million people, how many people aged 45 and over would probably have died from liver disease in 1990? Show your working. *(2 marks)*

  (ii)   Describe the trend in deaths from chronic liver disease for females aged 25–44 years between 1970 and 2000. *(1 mark)*

 (iii)   Suggest an explanation for the different death rates from liver disease of males aged 45–64 years and males aged 25–44 years. *(2 marks)*

  (b)   A breathalyser is a device that when blown in to, gives blood alchohol readings from a person's breath. The use of the breathalyser is well established in this country.

India is considering introducing the three different makes of breathalyser (**1–3**) by comparing their read-outs of blood alcohol concentration with that determined from a blood sample. A forensic scientist performed the tests on five individuals (**A–E**).

The table shows the results of the investigation.

Make	Time after drinking 90 cm³ alcohol (minutes)	Blood alcohol concentration of individuals A, B, C, D and E (mg per 100 cm³ blood) as measured by breathalyser (X) and directly from blood (Y)									
		A		**B**		**C**		**D**		**E**	
		X	**Y**	**X**	**Y**	**X**	**Y**	**X**	**Y**	**X**	**Y**
1	0	0	0	0	0	0	0	0	0	0	0
	30	47	22	53	21	27	9	29	7	47	22
	60	39	22	39	11	33	9	31	11	36	18
	90	33	26	37	12	22	11	25	11	32	18
2	0	0	0	0	0	0	0	0	0	0	0
	30	66	22	27	11	33	8.8	42	11	54	18
	60	50	22	60	12	33	9	42	11	54	18
	90	47	26	54	13	31	11	43	11	41	18
3	0	0	0	0	0	0	0	0	0	0	0
	30	68	22	84	21	41	9	41	7	85	22
	60	58	22	59	12	41	9	44	11	67	18
	90	50	26	57	13	34	11	44	11	52	18

(i) In general, how did the results for the breathalysers compare with the results directly from blood? *(1 mark)*

(ii) Which of the two methods of measuring blood alcohol is the more reliable? Support your answer with data from the table. *(2 marks)*

(iii) Which breathalyser would you advise the police to use? Explain the reasons for your answer. *(2 marks)*

(iv) The results for the five individuals varied. Suggest *three* reasons for this. *(3 marks)*

(a) Accidents sometimes damage the nervous system.

The diagram shows a test that doctors uses to find if there is damage.

When the tendon is struck with the hammer, the receptor is stimulated and the lower leg moves forward if there is no damage to nerves.

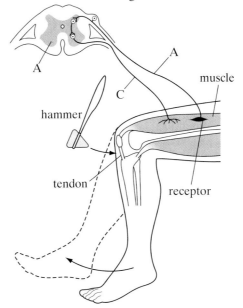

(i) Name the structures labelled **A**, **B** and **C**. *(3 marks)*

(ii) How is information passed from structure **A** to structure **B**? *(1 mark)*

(iii) What is the effector in this response? *(1 mark)*

(b) Every year at least 700 people in Britain break their back or their neck. This damages the spinal cord and may result in permanent paralysis.

The pie chart shows the causes of damage to the spinal cord.

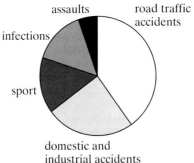

(i) Which is the commonest cause of damage to the spinal cord? *(1 mark)*

(ii) Calculate the proportion of injuries to the spinal cord caused by sport. *(1 mark)*

(c) Explain why a man with a damaged spinal cord cannot feel a pin stuck in his toe. *(3 marks)*

4 The diagram shows a cross-section through a human eye.

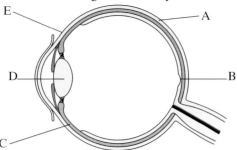

(a) Name the parts labelled **A**, **B**, **C**, **D** and **E**. *(5 marks)*

The drawing shows the structures in the human eye involved in focusing.

(b) Explain how the lens and structures **X** and **Y** enable a person to focus on distant objects.

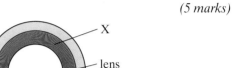

(3 marks)

5 Short-sighted people cannot focus clearly on distant objects. One way of correcting this condition is to use laser surgery to alter slightly the shape of the cornea. The diagram shows the effect of laser surgery on the shape of the cornea.

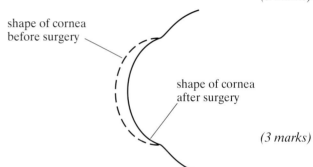

(a) Explain how laser surgery can correct short-sightedness. *(3 marks)*

(b) Look at the following safety poster.

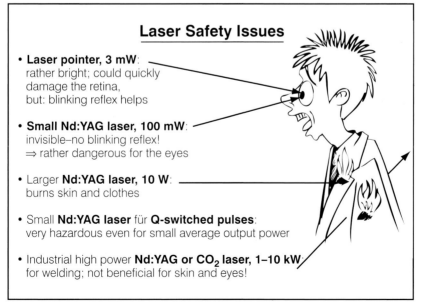

    (i)   On what does the amount of damage to the body caused by a laser mainly depend? *(1 mark)*

    (ii) What is meant by the blinking reflex? *(2 marks)*

    (iii) Explain why the blinking reflex cannot protect the eye from a small Nd:YAG laser. *(2 marks)*

6   Hormones control many processes in our bodies.

    (a) Copy the boxes below, and draw a straight line from each hormone to its function. *(4 marks)*

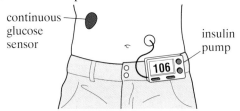

| Adrenaline |
| Oestrogen |
| Testosterone |
| Thyroxine |

| Controls male sexual development |
| Increases the heart rate during stress |
| Lower blood sugar levels |
| Controls metabloic rate |
| Controls female sexual development |

    (b) Describe the role of glucagon in the control of blood glucose concentration. *(3 marks)*

    (c) The drawing shows an 'artifcial pancreas'.

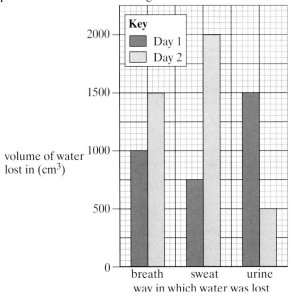

continuous glucose sensor

insulin pump

106

An artificial pancreas is a 'negative feedback' device that would regulate glucose levels in the body of someone with diabetes by continuously measuring the level of glucose and dispensing doses of insulin based on those measurements. An artificial pancreas would enable a person with diabetes to maintain 'normal' glucose levels by providing the right amount of insulin at the right time, just as a pancreas does in people without the disease.

    (i)   Explain what is meant by 'negative feedback'. *(2 marks)*

    (ii) Evaluate the use of an 'artificial' pancreas compared with the conventional treatment for diabetes. *(5 marks)*

7   The bar chart shows the amount of water lost from the body of a student on two different days.

The student ate the same amount of food and drank the same amount of liquid on the two days. The temperature of the surroundings was similar on the two days.

Key
■ Day 1
□ Day 2

volume of water lost in (cm³)

2000
1500
1000
500
0

breath   sweat   urine

way in which water was lost

(a) The total volume of water lost on Day 1 was $3250\,cm^3$.

How much water was lost on Day 2? Show all your working. *(2 marks)*

(b) The student did much more exercise on one of the days than on the other.

On which day did he do more exercise? Give *two* reasons for your answer. *(2 marks)*

(c) How does sweating help the body? *(1 mark)*

(d) Sports physiologists advise athletes how to cope with different climatic conditions.

Big athletes produce more heat and find it harder to keep cool. Shape matters too – a tall, thin runner has fewer problems keeping cool than a short, tubby runner of the same body mass. A 65 kg athlete running a marathon in 2 hours 10 minutes in reasonably dry conditions can avoid overheating at air temperatures up to 37 °C, but in humid conditions the same level of performance is possible only at temperatures below about 17 °C.

(i) Suggest why a 'tall, thin runner has fewer problems keeping cool than a short, tubby runner of the same body mass'. *(2 marks)*

(ii) Explain why runners are more likely to overheat in humid conditions. *(2 marks)*

8 We use muscles and bones for movement.

(a) The diagram shows the bones and some muscles in the wrist and hand of an adult human.

Use the diagram, together with your own knowledge of muscle action and the properties of muscles and tendons, to explain how the thumb and forefinger can grip and then release an object.

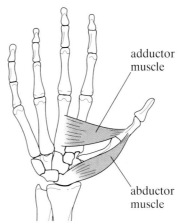

adductor muscle

abductor muscle

(3 marks)

(b) The diagram shows part of a human backbone.

(i) Give the normal function of the discs. *(1 mark)*

(ii) Describe *two* properties of cartilage which suit it to this function. *(2 marks)*

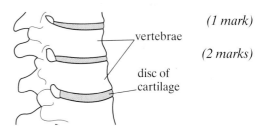

vertebrae

disc of cartilage

(c) Occupational therapists advise workers how to avoid occupational injuries.

Many people now use laptops at work.

Diagram 1 shows a man using a laptop placed on his desk. Diagram 2 shows the same man who has been advised by an occupational therapist to use his laptop on a stand.

Explain as fully as you can why using the laptop stand rather than placing the laptop on his desk is better for the man's health. *(3 marks)*

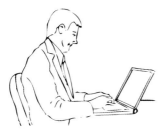

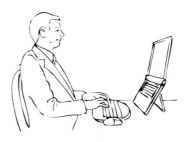

Diagram 1   **Diagram 2**

9.1   The human reproduction system

You started life as a single cell which was the result of your mother's **egg** being fertilised by your father's **sperm**. The male reproductive system is designed to produce millions of these sperm and to transfer them close to an egg. The function of the female reproductive system is to produce eggs, receive the sperm and allow the fertilised egg to develop into a baby.

Objectives

How do the reproductive organs work?

How are eggs and sperm different from other cells?

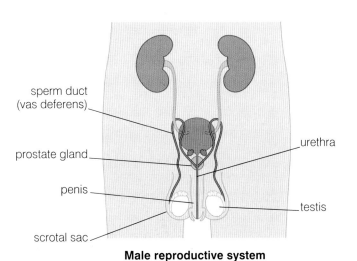

sperm duct (vas deferens)

prostate gland

penis

scrotal sac

urethra

testis

Male reproductive system

Male structure	Function
Penis	transfers semen (sperm plus seminal fluid) from male to female
Urethra	tube in penis which carries the semen
Testis	produces sperm and hormones
Scrotal sac	holds testes outside body to keep sperm 2 °C below body temperature
Sperm duct	carries sperm from testes to urethra
Prostate gland	produces seminal fluid

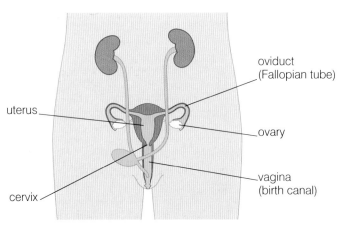

uterus

cervix

oviduct (Fallopian tube)

ovary

vagina (birth canal)

Female reproductive system

Female structure	Function
Ovary	produces eggs and hormones
Oviduct (Fallopian tube)	cilia in the lining of the tube waft the egg from the ovary to the unterus
Uterus	muscular wall protects the fetus, lining enables exchange of materials
Cervix	neck of the uterus, dilates during labour
Vagina (birth canal)	receives sperm and baby leaves body here

A *The male and female reproductive systems and the functions of the various structures*

Sex cells

Both the sex cells are called **gametes**. An egg and a sperm can be seen in Photo **B**. There are obvious differences in size and shape. These differences are due to the specialised nature of both the gametes. The sperm is small and has a tail to swim to the egg. The head of the sperm is filled by the nucleus. The egg also contains a nucleus, but its size is due to the presence of stored food.

Both cells have a nucleus but, unlike other body cells which have two sets of **23 chromosomes**, eggs and sperm only have one set. Eggs and sperm are produced by a method of cell division called **meiosis**, where cells with two sets of chromosomes divide to produce cells with one set (see page 78).

Fertilisation occurs when the nucleus of one sperm fuses with the nucleus of the egg. The **fertilised egg** (also called a **zygote**) will therefore have two sets or 23 pairs of chromosomes.

The fertilised egg divides into two cells, with identical sets of chromosomes, by a process called **mitosis**. These cells then divide many times to form a ball of identical cells or an embryo.

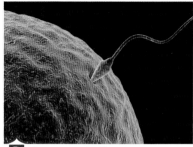

B   *Sperm penetrating an egg*

Did you know

After fertilisation the early fetus is called an embryo. Removing embryo cells and culturing them is one method of producing stem cells.

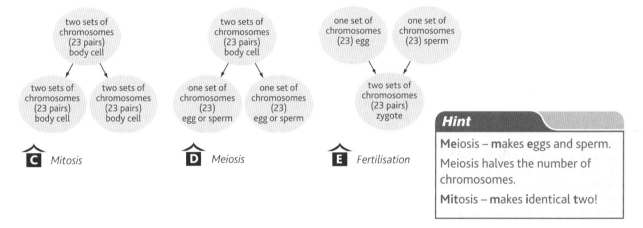

C   *Mitosis*

D   *Meiosis*

E   *Fertilisation*

Hint

Meiosis – makes **e**ggs and sperm.
Meiosis halves the number of chromosomes.
Mitosis – makes **i**dentical **t**wo!

Apply what you know

Embryos can be used as a source of stem cells. An egg is fertilised by a sperm in the laboratory and the cells divide for a few days. Cells are removed from this early embryo and provided with the conditions needed to multiply.

Adult stem cells can also be grown by selecting cells from human tissue. Scientists have to stimulate the stem cells to turn them into cells such as muscle, nerve or bone. It is hoped that stem cells will be used to replace damaged and diseased tissue.

1   Explain why eggs or sperm cannot be used as stem cells.

2   Which type of cell division takes place when stem cells multiply?

3   Some people disagree with using embryo stem cells. Suggest why.

In 2008 doctors transplanted part of a windpipe into a woman. Stem cells from the woman were used to produce new windpipe tissues on the donor organ.

4   What is the advantage of using adult stem cells in this way?

5   Scientists are still a long way from producing complete organs such as a heart. Suggest reasons for this.

Fertilisation

Fertilisation of the egg by the sperm takes place in the upper part of the **oviduct**. This means that the sperm have to swim there. Sperm are transferred from the male to the female during sexual intercourse. The penis becomes erect due to blood entering large blood spaces in the tissue, allowing the male to place the penis into the vagina. Semen travels through the urethra and is deposited very close to the cervix.

The area in and around the cervix is covered by mucus which can be very thick. When an egg has been released from the ovary (**ovulation**) in the middle of the **menstrual cycle** (see page 74) this mucus becomes more watery, making it easier for the sperm to enter the uterus and swim towards the oviduct. Millions of sperm are deposited, but only a few thousand reach the egg.

The egg is a large cell and is moved along by cilia on the oviduct surface. Only one sperm will penetrate the egg to form a zygote.

Twins

If two eggs are released from the ovary, and both are fertilised by separate sperm, twins will develop. These are **fraternal twins** and will be no more alike than any brothers and sisters.

The zygote divides into a ball of cells and moves down the oviduct to the uterus where some extraordinary changes take place in the ball. The embryo becomes embedded in the uterus lining (implantation) and layers of cells develop in the embryo which begins the development of the various body systems. Two other structures are also formed, the **placenta** and the **amnion**. Occasionally the embryo splits into two groups of cells at this stage and each develops into a separate fetus resulting in **identical twins**.

Changes to the uterus

Diagram **A** shows the fetus in the uterus after the amnion and placenta have developed. The amnion is a sac containing **amniotic fluid**. The fluid acts as a shock absorber to prevent damage to the fetus when the mother moves around.

You can see that the placenta penetrates the uterus lining. It acts as an exchange surface, enabling materials to pass between the fetus and the mother by **diffusion**, but keeps both bloodstreams separate.

Oxygen and soluble nutrients, e.g. glucose, amino acids, minerals and vitamins, diffuse from the mother's blood to the fetus. Carbon dioxide and other waste materials diffuse in the opposite direction. The umbilical cord contains blood vessels to transport the fetal blood between the fetus and placenta.

The **placenta** acts as a barrier to prevent large molecules and blood cells from passing to the fetus. Unfortunately, viruses such as those which cause rubella and HIV, are very tiny and can get across causing damage to the fetus. Rubella infection early in pregnancy can result in

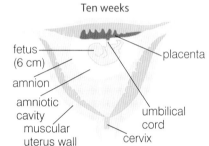

Ten weeks

A Fetus in the uterus in early stage of pregnancy

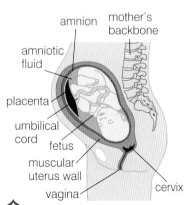

B Fetus in the uterus at late stage of pregnancy

miscarriage, still birth or birth defects such as deafness, cataracts or brain damage. This is rare in the UK now that most girls are vaccinated against rubella.

Midwives advise expectant mothers about diet and lifestyle during routine check-ups. Most would suggest that all women stop smoking, drink very little alcohol and always check with a doctor about taking medication.

Alcohol, drugs and chemicals from cigarettes can also cross the placenta and cause harm to the development of the fetus. Alcohol may cause learning difficulties by damaging the developing brain. The carbon monoxide from cigarettes reduces the oxygen available for aerobic respiration. There is less energy for growth resulting in babies with low birth weight.

Midwives also attend the birth, providing help, advice and essential drugs to support the mother through labour. Health visitors, or public health nurses, continue this work by monitoring the development of children, often in the home, and giving support and health advice to their parents.

Labour

Labour occurs in three main stages:

1   The muscular walls of the uterus contract in order to dilate (open up) the cervix.
2   The uterus walls squeeze to force the baby through the birth canal (vagina).
3   Following the birth the uterus contracts to push out the placenta.

Often the midwife will put the baby to the mother's breast as soon as it is born. This can help the delivery of the placenta and starts the suckling reflex in the baby. The first 'milk' contains a lot of antibodies which help to protect the baby from infections, but after a few days the milk will provide protein, fat and sugar in the correct proportions.

Human babies are totally dependent on their parents to care for them.

Foul facts

The nicotine in cigarettes causes blood vessels to go into spasm so the placenta receives less oxygen and nutrients. Nicotine reaching the fetus damages developing nerve cells and the brain. Cigarettes also contain other toxins which may harm the fetus.

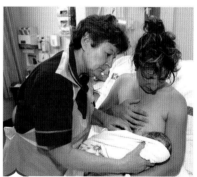

C   *A mother breastfeeds her newborn for the first time*

Apply what you know

1   Why is it dangerous if the mother's blood mixes with the blood of the fetus?

2   During pregnancy the lifestyle of the mother can have an impact on the developing fetus.

Why is it important that the mother has a healthy diet? Think about the energy and protein needed by the fetus for growth, the iron to make haemoglobin for red blood cells and the calcium for developing bones.

3   The mother also requires rest as well as moderate exercise. Moving helps to promote good circulation.

Why do you think an expectant mother needs rest?

4   What must parents do for a newborn baby?

Did you know ??????

Midwives and doctors recommend that babies are exclusively breastfed for six months to give them a healthy start. Formula milk is made to be as close to breast milk as possible.

Did you know ??????

Many animals care for their offspring, but this lasts longest in humans – over 30 years in some cases!

10 Human growth and development

10.1 Growth and puberty

Newborn babies grow at a very fast rate (see Graph **A**). In its first couple of months a baby may increase in size at about 2.5–4 cm per month and will continue to grow rapidly up to the age of 2. The rate of growth then steadies until **puberty,** when the young person has another growth spurt. During the early years of life the limbs will lengthen at a faster rate than the head and other organs grow. This means that the body proportions change.

Look at Diagram **B** and compare the youngest and oldest person. The head of the newborn is about one-quarter the length of its body, whereas the 25-year-old has a head that is approximately one-eighth of body length.

Objectives

How does your growth rate change?

How is society affected when large numbers of babies are born?

What is the menstrual cycle?

How are birth rates controlled?

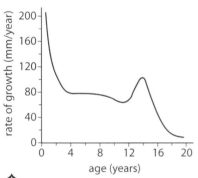
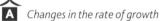

A *Changes in the rate of growth*

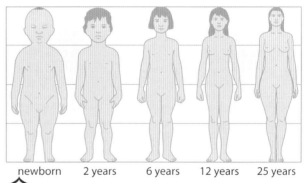

B *Postnatal body proportion changes*

Puberty

The age of starting puberty varies but averages around 12 years for girls and is usually earlier in girls than boys.

The changes which happen during puberty are controlled by the sex hormones, **oestrogen** and **testosterone**. These include changes in body shape, growth, voices and body hair as well as sperm production in boys and the start of menstruation (periods) in girls.

Menstrual cycle

For a girl, the first sign of puberty is when she has her first period. This loss of blood is the end of her first **menstrual cycle** and signals the beginning of her next cycle. Each cycle lasts approximately 28 days but can vary from 21 to 36 days. **Ovulation** (see page 72) occurs in the middle of the cycle. Because the cycle is controlled by hormones it is possible to stop the release of an egg by taking the hormone oestrogen in contraceptive pills.

Did you know ??????

At birth the brain is about 25% of the adult size. At age 7 it is 90%.

Did you know ??????

Puberty is generally a term used for the development of the secondary sexual characteristics – the physical changes that take place in the body.

Adolescence overlaps with puberty and includes all the psychological, behavioural and emotional changes in the teenage years.

Birth rate, fertility and contraception

How science works

In 2007 the British government warned that the current rise in the World population was unsustainable. Ministers proposed that use of contraceptive pills and the condom to reduce birth rate should be high on the agenda of countries where this is rising, to alleviate the problem of global poverty, starvation and possibly global warming.

In many countries, there are cultural and religious reasons why people think that artificial family planning methods are wrong because they interfere with the natural cycle. These could include:

- **contraception** where the egg is prevented from meeting the sperm, or implantation is prevented
- fertility treatment where the ovary is stimulated to produce extra eggs and there may be 'spare' embryos.

Natural methods of avoiding pregnancy can be used. Around ovulation the cervical mucus changes, the body temperature goes up by 0.5°C, and some women feel a slight abdominal ache. This means a woman can avoid having intercourse at the time of ovulation.

Discuss some of these issues with other people. Should governments insist that families can only have one child? Are natural methods likely to reduce the birth rate? What will happen in the future if the birth rate is lower than the death rate?

C   *Contraceptives: condoms and the contraceptive pill*

Sitting higher tier

Puberty starts when the **pituitary gland** is stimulated by chemicals, from the **hypothalamus**, and releases follicle stimulating hormone (FSH) and luteinising hormone (LH). These hormones reach the ovaries or testes, which in turn start to secrete **oestrogen** or **testosterone**. The increase in these hormones results in the development of the adult sexual characteristics.

Apply what you know

Graph **A** shows changes in the rate of growth from birth to age 20.

Use your knowledge and the graph showing growth rate at different ages to answer the questions.

1. Describe the shape of the graph.

2. The data for the graph was obtained by measuring growth rate in a large number of boys and girls.

   In what way is the data misleading about growth rate in:
   a   an individual
   b   in boys?

3. Suggest how the original data was recorded.

4. What useful information could you get from the original data which is not shown on the graph?

5. Suggest one change to make the graph more informative.

6. What type of graph/chart could be used to show all the original data?

10.2 Menstrual cycle

Sitting higher tier

Hormonal control of the menstrual cycle

This is a good example of negative feedback where production of one hormone can inhibit (switch off) the stimulating hormone.

There are four main hormones controlling the menstrual cycle.

- **FSH** stimulates follicles (egg-containing sacs) in the ovary to grow and to produce oestrogen.
- **LH** stimulates the release of the egg from the follicle at ovulation and the development of the corpus luteum, which is a yellow (luteum) body (corpus) formed by cells in the follicle after ovulation.
- **Oestrogen** causes the uterus lining to build up prior to ovulation.
- **Progesterone**, produced by the corpus luteum after ovulation, maintains the uterus lining ready for a fertilised egg.

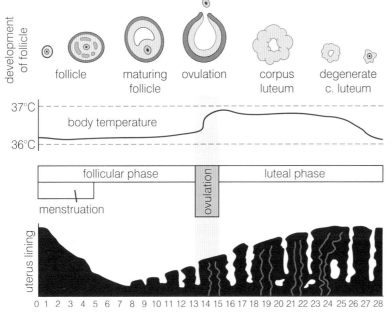

A *Diagram showing what happens to the follicle and uterus during the menstrual cycle*

The rising oestrogen levels between days 4–14 enter the bloodstream and stimulate the release of LH. The LH stimulates ovulation and causes the corpus luteum to produce progesterone. At the same time, the high level of oestrogen inhibits the production of FSH and more LH by the pituitary gland.

If the egg is fertilised it continues to travel down the oviduct and embeds in the uterus lining (see page 72). In this case, the oestrogen and progesterone continue to maintain the lining until 12 weeks into the pregnancy when the placenta produces enough progesterone to do this.

Objectives

How is the menstrual cycle controlled?

What part do hormones play in controlling the menstrual cycle?

How is infertility treated?

AQA Examiner's tip

Revise the section on hormones (7.3) before studying the menstrual cycle hormones.

Did you know ??????

Infertility treatments

- Specific hormone treatment can be used to treat women producing low hormone levels.
- IVF (in vitro fertilisation) uses hormones to stimulate the ovaries into developing follicles and release the eggs. These are collected by a doctor and fertilised in the laboratory. After a few days the embryos are screened and one is returned to the uterus to continue development. Some women suffer side effects from the high levels of hormones given.
- IVM (in vitro maturation) does not use high levels of hormones, immature eggs are collected from the ovary and matured in the laboratory before being fertilised. IVM is cheaper, takes less time and is safer for women than IVF.
- In vitro is Latin for within glass.

If implantation does not occur, then the ovary stops producing oestrogen and progesterone and the corpus luteum degenerates. The uterus lining breaks down resulting in the next period. The decreased level of oestrogen stops the inhibition of the pituitary gland and it releases FSH again.

Look for the links between hormones in Diagram **B**:

- Increasing FSH is followed by increasing oestrogen.

- Increasing oestrogen results in a sudden rise in LH.

- While combined oestrogen and progesterone are high the level of FSH is reduced.

B *Changes in hormone levels during the menstrual cycle*

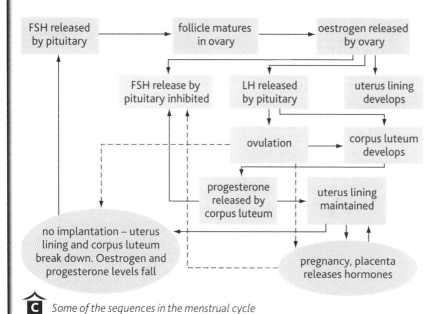

C *Some of the sequences in the menstrual cycle*

Cycle length	Probable ovulation day
25	11
26	12
29	15
30	16
31	17
35	21

Apply what you know

Use the graphs, diagrams and data in this chapter to answer the questions below:

1. Why are high doses of oestrogen given in contraceptive pills?

2. Some women miscarry around 12 weeks of pregnancy due to producing insufficient placental hormones. Which hormone may be given to prevent the breakdown of the uterus lining?

3. Which hormone(s) are given to a woman who is not ovulating or is undergoing egg collection, during **in vitro fertilisation treatment (IVF)**, which helps infertile women to have babies?

4. When women undergo IVF treatment, the eggs collected are fertilised by her partner's sperm in the laboratory and one embryo is implanted into the uterus. When is the best time to collect the eggs?

5. What are the advantages and disadvantages of IVF and IVM treatment?

6. Many women do not have 28 day cycles. If their periods are regular they can calculate their ovulation day by counting 14 days back from the next period. The table above shows some examples. What is the likely ovulation day for a woman with a 33 day cycle?

11.1 Inheritance of characteristics

In Chapter 9 you found out that 23 pairs of chromosomes are found in most human cells and that the two sets were brought together when the sperm fertilised the egg. This means that you inherit one set of chromosomes from each of your parents. Each chromosome contains a molecule called **DNA** (deoxyribonucleic acid). The DNA is divided along its length into hundreds of regions or genes, so you inherit half your **genes** from each parent.

Cell division and chromosomes

In Chapter 9 you learned that there are two types of cell division. The zygote divides by **mitosis** to give two genetically identical cells and all new body cells which are needed for growth and repair are formed by mitosis.

When gametes are produced each cell divides into four by **meiosis**. The gametes produced during meiosis are genetically different because there can be a variety of combinations of the chromosomes and there is also some exchange of alleles between them. This is why brothers and sisters have many similarities but are not identical.

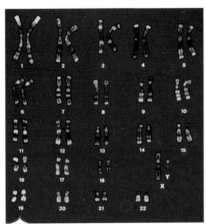

A *Human male chromosomes*

Look at the human chromosomes in Photo **A**, you will notice that 22 of the pairs are the same size and shape. The 23rd pair are labelled X and Y and are not the same. This indicates that the chromosomes are from a male and the Y chromosome has different genes from the X. Human females have two X chromosomes. This difference is significant at fertilisation. All eggs must have an X chromosome, but sperm may have an X or Y. So at fertilisation the **zygote** may be XX (female) or XY (male).

Visible changes in chromosomes are called chromosome **mutations**. Loss of a chromosome is usually fatal, because so many genes are missing. Duplication of the whole or part of a chromosome can lead to syndromes (groups) of disorders.

Objectives

What are chromosomes?

Why are gametes genetically different?

How are characteristics and genetic disorders inherited?

What are sex-linked genes?

Why are mutations harmful?

Find out ...

In the condition called Down's syndrome the person has an extra chromosome 21.

Find out how this extra chromosome affects the person's characteristics. You will realise that there is a range of features, because each individual will have different combinations of genes.

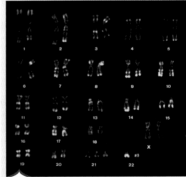

B *Chromosomes of someone with Down's syndrome*

What do genes do?

Every gene works as a **chemical code** instructing the cell to produce a particular protein. The protein may be an enzyme or other proteins which form structures in the body. If both your parents have blue eyes, you will inherit genes to make proteins which cause the iris to be blue. If one of your parents has brown eyes, you may have blue or brown eyes depending on the combination of genes you inherit.

On matching sites of the pairs of chromosomes the genes control the same protein. The 'matching' genes are referred to as **alleles,** so the genes for blue and brown eyes are alleles.

Accidental changes in the DNA structure are called **gene mutations.** Many characteristics, both normal and faulty, are the result of mutations which may have occurred many generations ago.

Sitting higher tier

A gene mutation can result in the loss of an enzyme or structural protein. If key cell reactions do not take place, a genetic disorder may occur; but some mutations have minor effects and may not be noticeable.

Foul facts

Several kings beheaded their wives for not producing sons to inherit the throne.

This was hardly fair, when it was the 'fault' of the king himself; it's the sperm that determine the baby's gender.

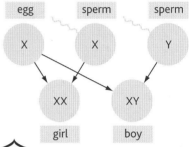

C *There is a 50% chance of having a boy or a girl at each fertilisation*

Scientists@work

Genetic counsellors

Cystic fibrosis (CF) is a genetically inherited disorder where the person produces very sticky mucus. CF is caused by a mutated gene on chromosome 7 (see Photo **A**). If the person inherits two of these alleles they will have cystic fibrosis. But people with one CF allele and one allele which has not mutated will produce normal mucus. We refer to the CF allele as **recessive**, because two copies are needed to have the disorder.

Huntington's disease is also an inherited disorder, causing degeneration of brain cells, but the symptoms do not usually show until the person is 30–50 years old. Only one copy of the faulty allele, found on chromosome 4, is needed to cause the condition. The allele is described as **dominant**, because it masks the effect of the 'normal' allele.

Genetic counsellors are able to advise people who suspect they may have inherited an allele for a genetic disorder, by working out the chances of their children having the condition. This is particularly important where the symptoms may not appear in the parent until the children have been born. Nowadays it is possible to identify the genes on the chromosomes and scientists can tell if the CF or Huntington's disease allele is faulty.

Physical characteristic are referred to as the **phenotype** and the genes you have as the **genotype.** The genotype is shown as letters, using a capital for the dominant gene. So a person with the phenotype cystic fibrosis must be **cc** and their parents would be **Cc**.

A person with Huntington's disease is usually **Hh** but, very rarely, could be **HH** if both parents had the condition.

Before working out inheritance of these fairly rare conditions, look at how a characteristic like eye colour can be inherited. Brown is dominant (**B**) to blue (**b**). Someone with brown eyes could be **BB** or **Bb**, but a person with blue eyes must be **bb**. If both alleles are the same we say the genotype is **homozygous,** so **BB** and **bb** are homozygous. **Bb** is described as **heterozygous,** because the alleles are different.

Suppose a father is homozygous for brown eyes and the mother has blue eyes, what colour eyes will their children have?

All their children will have brown eyes, because they can only inherit the allele for brown eyes from the father and the mother can only pass on an allele for blue.

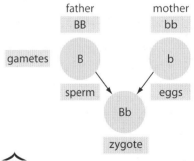
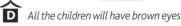

D *All the children will have brown eyes*

Punnett Squares

What are the chances of having blue eyes if the father is Bb (heterozygous) or both parents are Bb?

The easiest way to show this is on a diagram called a **Punnett square**.

father	mother
brown eyes	blue eyes
Bb	bb

		male gametes	
		B	b
	b	Bb brown	bb blue
female gametes	b	Bb brown	bb blue

E *In this case there is a 50:50 chance of a child having blue eyes*

father	mother
brown eyes	brown eyes
Bb	Bb

		male gametes	
		B	b
	B	Bb brown	Bb brown
female gametes	b	Bb brown	bb blue

F *In this case there is a 25% chance of a child having blue eyes. If there are four children in the family each child has a 25% chance of having blue eyes. By pure chance all could have brown eyes*

If you use the same principles but different letters you can work out any genetic cross.

Diagram **G** shows how the genetic counsellor can show two people without cystic fibrosis why their child inherited the disorder.

Remember that Huntington's disease is caused by a dominant gene. If a woman with the disease has children with a non-sufferer, then there is a 50% chance that each child could inherit it. See diagram **I**.

Practical activity

Genetics problems

You should be able to complete a Punnett square for new situations. Practise using other characteristics, e.g. having dimples (D) is dominant to no dimples (d); the ability to roll your tongue (R) is dominant to non-rolling (r).

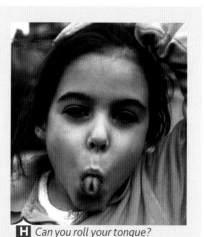

H *Can you roll your tongue?*

Find out ...

Genetics is a very important reason why we all have similar, but varied, characteristics; but other things can change our appearance. Differences in diet, the amount of exercise, whether we dye or perm our hair are all things which change us. Can you think of others?

Did you know ??????

Eye colour is actually controlled by several pairs of alleles, so don't worry if your eyes are not identical to either of your parents! Different combinations of genes can give all sorts of eye colours.

father	mother
non-sufferer	non-sufferer
Cc	Cc

		male gametes	
		C	c
	C	Cc non-sufferer	Cc non-sufferer
female gametes	c	Cc non-sufferer	cc cystic fibrosis

G *In this case there is a 25% chance of a child having cystic fibrosis*

father	mother
non-sufferer	Huntington's
hh	Hh

		male gametes	
		h	h
	H	Hh Huntington's disease	Hh
female gametes	h	hh non-sufferer	hh non-sufferer

I *In this case there is a 50% chance of a child having Huntington's disease*

AQA Examiner's tip

You will be expected to **construct** a Punnett square from information in the exam question.

Sitting higher tier

Sex-linked genes

In all the examples of inheritance described above the alleles are on chromosomes other than the X or Y. Y chromosomes are short and only have a few genes which are related to maleness. The X chromosome has many genes, which can only have alleles on the other X chromosome in a female.

Generally this is not a problem for males, but unfortunately there are some genes on the X chromosome which cause disorders:

■ colour blindness

■ haemophilia – a disorder where the blood does not clot properly

■ muscular dystrophy – a disorder where the muscles gradually degenerate.

If a boy has an X chromosome with the mutated allele, he will have the disorder even though it is recessive. If a girl has one faulty allele, she will also have a normal dominant allele on the other X chromosome and won't develop the disorder.

These genes are described as **sex-linked**. Diagram **J** shows how a boy can inherit colour blindness from his mother who has normal colour vision. The allele is shown attached to the X chromosome (X^c).

	father	mother
	normal vision	normal vision
	XY	X^c X

		male gametes	
		X	Y
female gametes	X^c	X^c X carrier girl	X^c Y colour blind boy
	X	XX normal vision girl	XY normal vision boy

J *It is possible to have a colour blind girl. Can you work out the genotypes of her parents? Remember she needs to inherit two alleles for colour blindness.*

Did you know ??????

Fathers cannot pass a sex-linked disorder to their sons because boys inherit the Y chromosome.

Cystic fibrosis

Cystic fibrosis can be detected by blood tests or high levels of salt in a newborn's sweat. It can be detected before birth by testing a sample of amniotic fluid (amniocentesis) or a biopsy of the placenta (chorionic villus sampling).

Cystic fibrosis is treated with physiotherapy, medication containing enzymes, antibiotics and, in severe cases, heart and lung transplants.

Scientists are investigating gene therapy as an alternative treatment.

Scientists@work

Apply what you know

1. The ability to roll the tongue is controlled by a dominant gene (R). A couple have two children, their son can roll his tongue but their daughter cannot do this. Both the parents can roll their tongues so are rather puzzled! They also want to know the probability of a third child being able to roll its tongue and the chances of having another son or daughter. How would you explain this to them? Use a Punnett square to help you.

2. Which parent determines the sex of the baby? Explain your answer.

3. Haemophilia is a sex-linked disorder. It normally affects boys, but can be inherited by girls in rare circumstances. Explain how this is possible.

AQA Examiner's tip

Always use 'alleles' not 'genes' when referring to a pair of alleles which control the same characteristic.

Did you know ??????

DNA stands for deoxyribose nucleic acid.

How science works

The development of genetic engineering was prompted by suggestions that the supplies of insulin from pigs and cows would run short by this century, due to more people living longer and developing diabetes. Pharmaceutical companies looked for other ways of producing large quantities of insulin and the science of **genetic engineering** was born. They discovered **specific enzymes** which could cut out the coding sequences of the insulin gene and were then able to transfer the gene to a ring of DNA called a **plasmid**, using other enzymes. Plasmids are found naturally in **bacteria** so the next step was to transfer the plasmids with the human insulin gene back into a common bacterium, *E.coli*.

Bacteria multiply rapidly, duplicating exact copies of the plasmids and then splitting into two – in a similar way to mitosis. This means that all the cells are genetically the same and their DNA will code for the production of the human insulin protein. Genetically identical cells are called **clones**.

Huge numbers of the cloned bacteria are grown in containers called fermenters, and each cell produces insulin. Eventually the cells are removed from the fermenter and the insulin is separated from the bacteria and purified.

This method produces insulin quickly, relatively cheaply and does not depend on removing the pancreas from pigs and cows. This is beneficial because some diabetics did not like using animal products for their treatment, and as the insulin is identical to human insulin there is also less chance of allergic reactions. Diagram **B** shows the process of genetic engineering.

Insulin is quite a small protein, so it was a good choice to start the technology. Now scientists are able to manufacture many products, including vaccines, by genetic engineering.

Objectives

What is genetic engineering?

What are the benefits of genetic engineering?

What is gene therapy?

What are stem cells?

What are the advantages and disadvantages of these therapies?

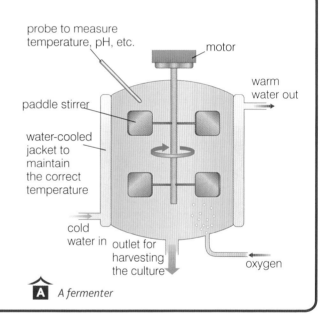

probe to measure temperature, pH, etc.

motor

warm water out

paddle stirrer

water-cooled jacket to maintain the correct temperature

cold water in

outlet for harvesting the culture

oxygen

A | *A fermenter*

Sitting higher tier

Gene therapy

Scientists are finding ways of correcting faulty genes to cure genetic disorders. The main problem is transferring the non-faulty gene to the appropriate cells. In some cases the 'carrier' used is a **virus** because they are small enough to enter cells. In 2008 scientists started clinical trials to test gene therapy treatments on patients with cystic fibrosis. Lung cells are difficult to target because lungs are designed to remove particles (see Chapter 5) and the person with CF produces very sticky mucus, so there have been many problems to overcome.

Another possibility is to screen very early embryos for the presence of a CF gene and replace it with the normal gene. This means that as the cells divide to form the fetus they will all contain the normal gene and the person will not have CF.

Foul facts

At one time human growth hormone was harvested from dead bodies.

FSH was purified from the urine of post-menopausal women.

The blood clotting factor VIII, needed by haemophiliacs, was collected from blood.

Now all these proteins are made by genetic engineering.

Stem cell therapy

For years doctors have been treating leukaemia (a form of cancer of the blood cells) with bone marrow from donors. In the bone marrow are cells called **stem cells** that replace the many blood cells which naturally die every day. These adult stem cells divide and can then change into different types of blood cells – they **differentiate**. During treatment, the patient's bone marrow is destroyed by chemotherapy and radiation, then the donor cells are put into the patient's blood. The cells migrate to the bone marrow and start dividing and differentiating.

In some cases the person's own bone marrow is removed, treated to kill the cancer cells and returned to the person, lowering the risk of rejection.

Current research on stem cells uses the same principle. Cells which have not differentiated are identified, collected and cultured in the laboratory. It is hoped to replace damaged tissue, e.g. nerves, muscles, pancreas etc., with these cultured cells. However it is important to realise that there are many complex mechanisms involved and the process is not as easy as it might sound. To make new nerve cells only the nerve cell genes must be 'switched on' in the stem cell.

Undifferentiated stem cells can also be collected from umbilical cord blood and from human embryos less than 14 days old. Cord blood could be collected and stored as a source of stem cells if needed by the person when they grow up.

- Using aborted embryos, or spare embryos from IVF treatment, is highly controversial.

- Try to explain the benefits of stem cells to someone who knows little biology and then discuss with them whether embryonic stem cells should be developed.

How science works

human cell with insulin gene in its DNA

bacterium with ring of DNA called plasmid

insulin gene cut out of DNA by an enzyme

plasmid taken out of bacterium and split open by an enzyme

insulin gene inserted into plasmid by another enzyme

plasmid with insulin gene in it taken up by bacterium

bacterium multiplies many times in fermenter

the insulin gene is switched on and the insulin is harvested from the bacteria

insulin

B *Nowadays all diabetics are treated with insulin from genetically engineered bacteria.*

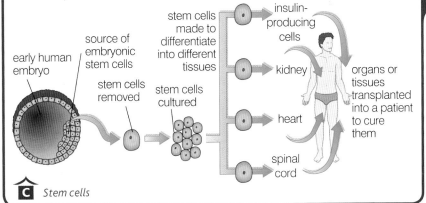

early human embryo

source of embryonic stem cells

stem cells removed

stem cells cultured

stem cells made to differentiate into different tissues

insulin-producing cells

kidney

heart

spinal cord

organs or tissues transplanted into a patient to cure them

C *Stem cells*

Apply what you know

1 What are the advantages of using genetically engineered bacteria to produce human proteins?

2 Suggest some of the conditions needed in the fermenter for bacterial growth and insulin production.

3 Changing genes in an embryo is a controversial idea. What are the pros and cons of this type of gene therapy?

4 What is the advantage of storing cord blood for an individual who may need it as an adult?

12.1 Pathogens and disease

Pathogens come in all shapes and sizes but most of them are only visible with microscopes so we call them **microbes** (or **microorganisms**). In fact there are thousands of microbes which are harmless and have important roles in nature. We depend on bacteria and fungi to decay all the dead plants and animals. Imagine what the world would be like if these just piled up! Unfortunately some microbes cause **infectious diseases** and these are referred to as pathogens.

There are four main groups of pathogen:

- viruses
- bacteria
- fungi
- protoctistans.

Viruses

Viruses (see Diagram **A**) are so small they can only be seen with the electron microscope. They are nature's 'genetic engineers' because they transfer their genes into the cells of other organisms. They have a protein coat and contain DNA or another similar chemical called **RNA** (ribonucleic acid). Viruses inject their DNA into body cells, which use the genes in the viral DNA to produce new viruses. These viruses are released and enter more body cells causing damage and setting up an immune response (see Chapter 13).

Common colds, influenza, measles, mumps, rubella and chicken pox are caused by viruses.

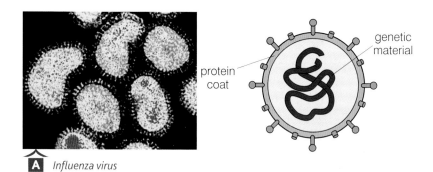

protein coat

genetic material

A *Influenza virus*

Treatment of viral infections

There are only a few antiviral drugs, so most of the treatment is with drugs to relieve the headaches, fevers or rashes which often occur with viral infections. Scientists have also produced many vaccines which prevent viral diseases (see Chapter 13).

Objectives

What causes disease?

How are diseases passed on?

How does lifestyle affect the spread of disease?

Foul facts

Your body contains about ten times as many bacteria as body cells! Don't worry though – most of them are in your gut and help to digest and make vital nutrients.

They also make smelly gases by breaking down food like baked beans.

Foul facts

Botulinum nerve toxin (Botox), from a bacterium, causes paralysis and is one of the most lethal toxins known. In a dilute form it is used to remove wrinkles.

Bacteria

Bacteria (Diagram **B**) are bigger than viruses and can be seen with the light microscope if they are stained to make them visible. Bacteria multiply rapidly and cause disease in two ways:

- direct damage to the body tissues
- production of toxins (poisons) which can go into the bloodstream and affect many parts of the body.

Salmonella food poisoning, MRSA, tuberculosis, pneumonia and cholera are caused by bacteria.

Treatment of bacterial infections

Bacteria can be killed by **antibiotics.** Doctors will often send a sample of blood to a microbiologist who will identify which bacterium is causing the disease. The doctor can then prescribe the specific antibiotic to kill that type of bacterium.

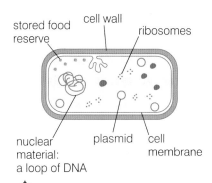

B A bacterium

Fungi

Fungi (Photo **C**) are not all as big as mushrooms! Some small fungi live on the surface of our skin, especially where it is warm and damp. Athlete's foot, thrush and ringworm are common fungal infections. The athlete's foot and ringworm appear as patches on the surface skin, but thrush (a yeast-like fungus) usually affects the skin lining the mouth or vagina. The natural bacteria in our bodies seem to prevent thrush from developing. It is more common in babies who do not have many bacteria and in people who have taken antibiotics.

Protoctistans

Protoctistans (Photo **D**) are a group of single-celled organisms, some of which cause disease. **Malaria** is still a major disease which kills millions of people and is caused by a protoctistan called plasmodium. People become infected when they are bitten by a mosquito (Photo **E**). The plasmodium is transferred into the person's blood and infects the liver and then the red blood cells. If another mosquito has a blood meal it picks up the plasmodium. We say that the mosquito acts as a **vector** of the disease.

Amoebic dysentery is an infection of the intestines, causing severe diarrhoea. The amoeba usually enters the body in contaminated food and drink and multiplies in the gut. Poor sanitation can cause the spread of the amoebae from the faeces of an infected person.

Treatment for fungal and protoctistan infections

There are antifungal creams and drugs, but it is best to avoid infection if possible for many of these diseases. Fungi are easy to pick up from other people in shared damp places, such as changing rooms. Malaria can be prevented by taking specific drugs, such as quinine and avoiding being bitten by the mosquito.

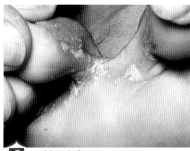

C Athlete's foot

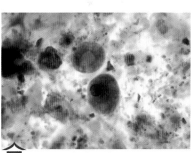

D Entamoeba histolytica

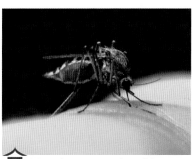

E Mosquitoes are carriers of the protoctistan which causes malaria

Transmission of disease

The most common ways in which disease is passed from one person to another is by **close contact**. This can be when directly touching infected skin or by transferring microbes when kissing or by sexual intercourse.

Coughing and sneezing while you are infected will spray drops of water containing huge numbers of viruses or bacteria into the air, which can be inhaled by other people. This is called **droplet infection**.

You have already learned about the importance of avoiding contaminated food and drink. Think of all the ways that bacteria may be transferred from infected people to food and remember that bacteria will multiply rapidly in warm conditions.

Houseflies as well as mosquitoes can act as vectors. They can carry bacteria on their bodies as they fly from unhygienic places to food.

AQA Examiner's tip

- Remember viruses need to reproduce in other cells.
- Bacteria divide into two to reproduce.
- Antibiotics only kill bacteria; they cannot be used to treat viruses.

How science works

Some facts about a cholera epidemic in Angola (Africa) in 2006

Scientists need to analyse information from a wide variety of sources in order to solve problems. Here are some facts about a cholera epidemic in Angola (Africa) in 2006.

Facts about cholera	Facts about the epidemic
• Cholera is a bacterial disease	• 35 000 people fell ill and 1200 died in the first three months of the outbreak
• The bacteria can be carried, for up to two weeks, in the faeces of people who do not become ill	• Half the sick were in the capital Luanda
• The bacteria live in dirty water	• The outbreak started in the slums of Luanda and spread to 11 of the 18 provinces
• The symptoms are diarrhoea and vomiting	
• Children and the elderly can become dehydrated	• Luanda's slums are crowded and lack adequate water and sanitation
• Clean water and re-hydration tablets are successful treatments	
• Travellers to Africa are usually offered oral vaccines	• People move about freely in Angola

Scientists@work

Louis Pasteur discovered that microbes made wine go bad. He developed the process of **pasteurisation** for wine and milk.

Both Pasteur and Robert Koch discovered the microbes which cause TB, anthrax, cholera and many other diseases.

Apply what you know

1 Use the information above to answer the questions:

a What was the likely cause of the cholera outbreak in Luanda?

b Why did the disease spread to the provinces?

c Who are the most likely people to die of cholera?

d Why is it difficult to treat cholera in Angola?

e What advice could you give to a Luandan to avoid becoming infected or passing the infection to someone else?

f How can outbreaks of cholera be prevented?

2 Why will taking antibiotics allow thrush to develop?

3 Can you suggest ways to avoid contracting:

a malaria

b amoebic dysentery?

4

a How can you reduce the spread of pathogens by droplet infection?

b How can you prevent food from being contaminated by *Salmonella*?

12.2 Defence against disease

Outer defences

The human body has several ways of preventing the entry of pathogens.

The **skin** which covers the body is designed to act as a barrier. The outer layer is made of dead cells and it prevents pathogens from reaching the cells beneath.

If bacteria are inhaled they are trapped by the mucus which lines the respiratory passages. This mucus is then wafted up by the **cilia** on the cells which line the trachea and bronchi and swallowed or coughed out.

Many pathogens are killed by the strong acid in the stomach, because the acid denatures the enzymes. Other tubes such as the vagina and urethra, which open to the external environment, also have acid secretions to kill some pathogens.

When you cut yourself the **blood clots** and forms a **scab** (see page 26), preventing the entry of pathogens. At the same time **white blood cells** surround the area to destroy any pathogens which might enter (see Chapter 13).

Precautions

Generally these protective mechanisms are very successful and we can also help ourselves by being 'bug aware'. Eating healthily, washing regularly, cleaning teeth, hygienic preparation of meals, maintaining clean kitchens and bathrooms will all reduce our contact with pathogens. Our drinking water is treated to remove particles by filtering and to kill microbes by adding chlorine to our water supply. It is also important that waste water from sinks and toilets is properly treated, at sewage works, to kill microbes.

Internal defences

Despite all these natural defences, and man-made precautions, we become ill when a large number of pathogens enter the body at the same time and continue to reproduce. Fortunately the body responds by detecting the foreign microbes and the white blood cells produce **antibodies** and **anti-toxins** to combat them (see Chapter 13). It takes a short time for the immune system to build up enough of these, and in the mean time we can suffer the symptoms of the disease.

On page 84 you learned that viruses are found inside the body cells and this makes them difficult to treat without damaging the cells too. In this case prevention is better than cure, so scientists have developed vaccines for many viral diseases.

Some bacteria damage cells, while others produce poisons. In the past, bacterial infections often proved fatal. Many soldiers died from infections of even minor wounds, and large numbers of women died following childbirth in hospitals due to doctors passing infection from one patient to the next.

Objectives

How does the body protect itself from pathogens?

How were antibiotics discovered?

Discovering antibiotics – 'Chance favours the prepared mind'

In 1928, **Alexander Fleming** made a chance observation which was to save millions of lives. Fleming was a trained doctor who was researching bacteria, when he returned from a holiday to find one of his bacterial culture plates left out on a window sill without the lid (see Photo **A**). He noticed that the bacteria were growing over the whole plate, except in a clear area around some mould. Fortunately Fleming realised the significance of his observation – a chemical in the mould was killing the bacteria. He cultured the *Penicillium* mould and performed more experiments to extract small quantities of the active substance, which he called **penicillin**. Although Fleming tested his penicillin on mice, little progress was made for ten years, as he continued with his other research.

Then two more scientists, **Florey**, a doctor, and **Chain**, a biochemist, working as part of a research team in Oxford, read Fleming's research paper on penicillin. They cultured various varieties of mould, selecting the one which produced most penicillin.

Florey and Chain went a step further than Fleming, by testing mice which had been deliberately infected with bacteria. Half the mice received penicillin and survived but the control group, without the drug, died. Then they tested it on a man with a serious infection. He recovered at first, but they could not finish his treatment and he died. However their initial success prompted pharmaceutical companies to provide money for further research and, eventually, large quantities of penicillin and other antibiotics were being produced. Doctors were now able to cure the majority of patients with bacterial infections.

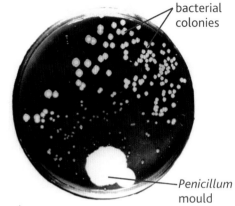

bacterial colonies

Penicillum mould

A Fleming's bacterial culture plate

Practical activity

PSA / ISA

You may have the opportunity to investigate the effect of antibiotics on different bacteria. Remember to work safely and measure accurately. Find out which antibiotics work best. Are all bacteria equally affected? What is the dependent variable?

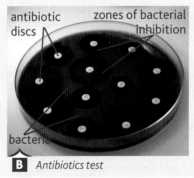

antibiotic discs

zones of bacterial inhibition

bacteria

B Antibiotics test

Apply what you know

Read the passage about discovering antibiotics and answer the questions:

1. If Fleming had been doing his research today it would be unlikely for the plate to become contaminated with mould. Suggest reasons for this.

2. Some people would have thrown away a mouldy plate. Why did Fleming keep his?

3. Suggest reasons for the success of Florey, Chain and their team.

4. What are the ethical issues connected with this research?

5. Why can't we treat viruses with antibiotics?

Did you know ??????

Fleming, Florey and Chain received the Nobel Prize for Medicine in 1945, but we must not forget that they worked with many other scientists to extract and develop penicillin.

12.3 Outbreak!

◼ Antibiotic resistance

For over 60 years doctors have been prescribing antibiotics which has led to a new problem in the battle against disease.

Antibiotics work by either damaging the wall of the bacterium or interfering with its growth mechanism. However, some bacteria have **mutations** which make them **resistant** to antibiotics – their walls are protected or they can continue to grow. Provided there are only a few of these mutant forms, the body's immune system can destroy them while the antibiotics work on the non-resistant bacteria. But if there are large numbers of the resistant bacteria in the body, the person can become ill and of course the antibiotics cannot kill the bacteria.

So how have large numbers of resistant-bacteria built up?

All organisms **compete** for food and space so very large numbers of bacteria compete with each other. Small numbers of mutant bacteria have to compete with the large numbers of non-resistant ones. But what happens if all the non-resistant ones disappear when we take antibiotics? No competition! The resistant forms multiply rapidly, using the food and space. We call this process **natural selection**. The non-resistant bacteria are killed by the antibiotics, the mutant, resistant, forms **survive** and reproduce.

Objectives

What is antibiotic resistance?

How can hospitals reduce the spread of infection?

colony of bacteria — antibiotic 1 — 95% of bacteria killed by antibiotic

5% survive – they have a mutation which makes them resistant to antibiotic 1

colony of bacteria resistant to antibiotic — antibiotic 2 — 95% of bacteria killed by antibiotic

colony of bacteria resistant to antibiotics 1 and 2... — antibiotic 3 — 5% survive – they have a mutation which makes them resistant to antibiotic 2 as well

A Bacteria can develop resistance to many different antibiotics

MRSA

Over-use of antibiotics has led to a rapid increase in bacteria which are resistant to antibiotics. Methicillin-resistant *Staphylococcus aureus* (**MRSA**) is an example which has been the subject of much media coverage. People who have open wounds or may be in poor health are particularly vulnerable to MRSA infection when in hospital.

Hospital infection control teams have worked hard to limit the problem. **Microbiologists** identify pathogens and suggest the appropriate control methods. Some methods are:

- provision of alcohol-based hand washes, for all staff and visitors to use
- improving basic hygiene on wards, since it was found that staff were inadvertently transmitting the bacteria on equipment such as stethoscopes and even pens used to write patients' notes
- ensuring ward furniture and equipment is cleaned with disinfectants and antiseptics to kill bacteria on the surfaces
- the occasional use of special paint containing chemicals to destroy bacteria.

Scientists@work

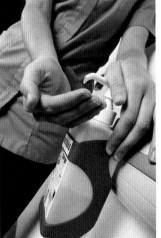

B An alcohol-based hand wash in a hospital

Did you know ??????

An epidemic occurs when large numbers of people have a disease. If the epidemic spreads to many countries it is called a pandemic.

Clostridium difficile

Another bacterium, *Clostridium difficile* or *C. diff.* is commonly found in the large intestine, surrounded by millions of natural, safe, bacteria. When antibiotics are prescribed many of the safe bacteria can be destroyed allowing the *C. diff.* to multiply, produce toxins and cause diarrhoea, a common side effect of antibiotic treatment.

C. diff produces spores which can survive in the environment and are not affected by alcohol washes. In recent years a more toxic type of *C. diff.* has been identified so hospital staff are told to wash hands with soap and water, to remove faecal contamination, and to clean toilets, sinks and floors in affected wards with bleach.

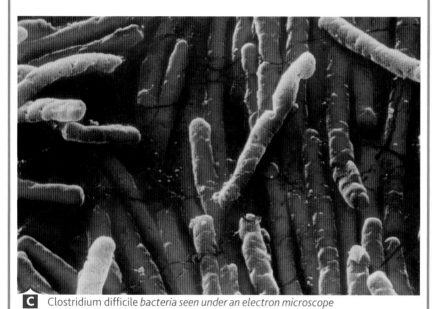

C Clostridium difficile *bacteria seen under an electron microscope*

Did you know ???????

The Health Protection Agency offers advice and oversees infection control in UK hospitals.

Remember

▦ Do not confuse antibiotics and antiseptics.

▦ Antibiotics kill bacteria inside the body.

▦ Antiseptics can only be used on the skin; they are dangerous if swallowed.

AQA Examiner's tip

Make sure you know how bacteria become resistant. Use the words competition, selection, survival and reproduction.

Apply what you know

1 Make a list of all the ways that diseases can be transmitted in hospitals – do not forget coughing or sneezing and think about what people do as they move around.

2 What advice would you give to the following people to help them control infection in a hospital: a member of the medical team, a patient, a ward orderly who serves the meals, and a cleaner?

Chapters 9–12

1 The diagram shows some parts of the male reproductive system.

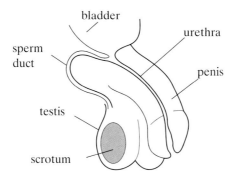

(a) What is the advantage of having the testes held outside the body in the scrotum? *(2 marks)*

(b) During intercourse, sperm must be moved from the testes along the sperm ducts and through the urethra. Just before the sperm enter the urethra, a number of secretions are added.

  (i) How are the sperm moved along the sperm ducts? *(1 mark)*

  (ii) What is the name of the mixture of sperm and the secretions which travels through the urethra? *(1 mark)*

(c) After intercourse, one sperm may fertilise an egg cell in one of the fallopian tubes. In fertilisation, the nucleus of the sperm enters the egg cell and fuses with the nucleus of the egg cell. The single cell which is formed is called a zygote.

  (i) In humans, how many chromosomes are there in:

    A the sperm

    B the egg cell

    C the zygote? *(3 marks)*

  (ii) How does the zygote become an embryo? *(1 mark)*

2 Health visitors advise mothers to breastfeed their babies.

(a) Give two reasons why breastfeeding is beneficial to babies. *(2 marks)*

(b) Research in 1929 showed a link between breast feeding and intelligence in babies; breast-fed babies tend to have a higher IQ than bottle-fed babies.

Read the following report of recent research into this link.

The researchers analysed data from more than 5000 children and 3000 mothers in the US.

They found that mothers who breastfed tended to be more intelligent, and when this fact was taken into account, most of the relationship between breastfeeding and the child's intelligence disappeared.

The rest was accounted for by other aspects of the family background.

The researchers also looked at families where one child was breastfed and another was not.

This confirmed the earlier results - the breastfed child was no more intelligent than his or her sibling.

Mr Der said: 'This research shows that intelligence is determined by factors other than breastfeeding.'

Rosie Dodds, of the National Childbirth Trust, said 'the study was not conclusive'.

She said a study in the Philippines - where, unlike the West, poorer women are more likely to breastfeed, showed that breastfed children were likely to be more intelligent.

However, she added: 'Women do not breastfeed because of any benefit to their baby, they do it because it feels like the natural thing to do.'

'It is important that women make a decision that is right for them, and their family, and they should not be pressurised either way, but we would like to see more support for women who do decide they want to breastfeed.'

Using information from the passage, evaluate the evidence for a link between breastfeeding and intelligence. *(5 marks)*

3   The diagram shows the relative sizes of different parts of the body of a newly born baby and of an adult.

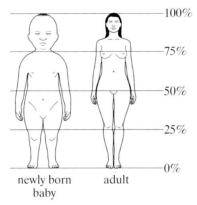

(a) In the newly born baby, about what proportion of the body consists of the head?   *(1 mark)*

(b) In the adult, about what proportion of the body consists of the head?   *(1 mark)*

(c) What happens to the relative rate of growth of the head and of the legs as a person grows up?   *(2 marks)*

Table 1 shows the age range at which various events in puberty occurred in a large sample of females and males.

Table 1

Event	Age range over which event occurred (years)
Height spurt (females)	9.5–14.5
Height spurt (males)	10.5–16.5
First menstrual period	10.5–16.0
Breasts start to develop	8.0–13.0
Rate of growth of penis increases	10.5–14.5
Rate of growth of testes increases	9.5–13.5

(d) Which hormone is mainly responsible for:

   (i)   the height spurt in both females and males?   *(1 mark)*

   (ii) the development of breasts?   *(1 mark)*

(e) From the information in the table:

   (i)   by what age had all the girls completed puberty?   *(1 mark)*

   (ii) by what age had puberty started in all the boys?   *(1 mark)*

4 (a) The graph shows the concentrations of two hormones during one sexual cycle of a human female. The diagram shows structures that produce these hormones.

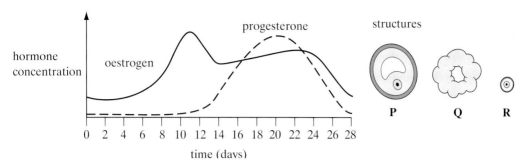

(i) Copy the graph and write the appropriate letters on it to show the order in which the structures labelled **P** to **R** appear during the cycle. *(1 mark)*

(ii) Name the hormone that causes structure Q to develop. *(1 mark)*

(b) Describe *two* effects of progesterone on the uterus. *(2 marks)*

(c) The graph shows the percentage of live births by age group and mean age of women at childbearing, for England and Wales, 1976–98.

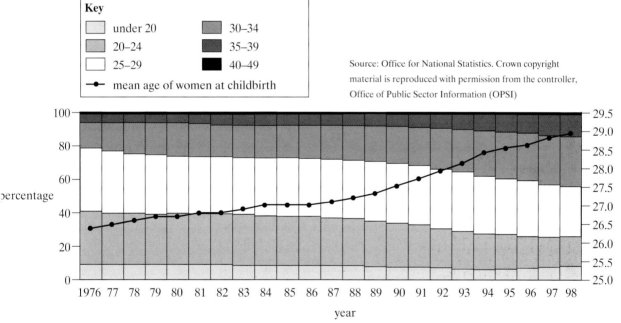

Source: Office for National Statistics. Crown copyright material is reproduced with permission from the controller, Office of Public Sector Information (OPSI)

(i) Describe the trends shown by the graph. *(2 marks)*

(ii) Suggest explanations for these trends. *(2 marks)*

5   A couple has just found out that the woman is pregnant. They wonder whether the child will be a boy or a girl.

(a) Write the sex chromosomes of the man and the woman.   *(2 marks)*

(b) The couple already has one girl. What is the chance that the new baby will be another girl?

Explain the reason for your answer. You may use a genetic diagram if you wish.   *(3 marks)*

Crigler-Najjar (C-N) syndrome is a rare genetic disorder controlled by a recessive allele. Individuals with the disorder are unable to break down bilirubin, a toxic waste product formed when the liver destroys old red blood cells. Children with this syndrome must sleep under special blue lights which destroy bilirubin. If this treatment fails a liver transplant is required.

(c) A genetic counsellor would advise parents on the chances of their child inheriting C-N syndrome.

Use a genetic diagram to show how two people, neither of whom shows the disorder, can have a child with C-N syndrome.   *(3 marks)*

(d) C-N syndrome is a very rare condition. The syndrome is common in one particular community. This community is described as closed as marriage occurs only between its members.

Suggest how C-N syndrome has become common in a closed community.   *(3 marks)*

(e) Recent studies have shown that it may be possible to repair the defective gene in the liver cells of affected individuals. Successful gene therapy of all individuals with this disorder in this community might increase the frequency of C-N syndrome in future generations. Suggest how this might happen.   *(2 marks)*

6   (a) (i) What is meant by a stem cell?   *(1 mark)*

    (ii) Stem cells divide by mitosis.

         Explain why cells produced by mitosis have identical genetic information. *(2 marks)*

(b) Haematologists are developing techniques using stem cells to treat blood disorders.

Read the passage below about stem cells and genetic screening.

A boy has been born to a British couple who want to use stem cells from hisumbilical cord to treat an older brother with a life threatening blood disorder.The disorder can only be cured by a transplant of stem cells from a sibling with a perfect tissue match.

Michelle and Jason Whitaker's baby, Jamie, was genetically selected while he was still an embryo to be a near perfect match to four-year-old Charlie. The couple went to an American clinic for test-tube baby treatment because the selection procedure is not allowed in the UK.

Mr Whitaker told the newspaper: 'All we did was change the odds from a one-in-four chance of a tissue match to almost 100%. There was no selection on the basis of colour of eyes, hair or sex.'

The Human Fertilisation and Embryology Authority said it was acceptable to test and select embryos to prevent the birth of a baby with a genetic disease, but not to select them in order to help another child.

But John Smeaton, national director of the Society for the Protection of Unborn Children, said: 'Human beings who were not the perfect match were simply discarded and a child has been created with the primary purpose of benefiting his elder brother.'

Use information from the passage to evaluate whether genetic screening should be allowed in cases similar to that of Jamie and Charlie.

Explain the reasons for your answer.   *(4 marks)*

7   Read the following passage about tuberculosis.

One of the deadliest diseases seems to be making a comeback in Britain. Doctors are alarmed at the rising number of cases of tuberculosis (TB).TB is caused by microbes called bacteria. When people carrying the TB bacteria cough or sneeze, the TB bacteria get into the air. Other people may then breathe them in.

(a) Which organs will be infected first when someone breathes in the TB bacteria?   *(1 mark)*

(b) Explain how the TB bacteria inside the body may cause disease.   *(2 marks)*

(c) Name *one other* group of microbes that often causes disease.   *(1 mark)*

(d) People who live in overcrowded areas are more likely to catch TB than people who live in less crowded areas. Suggest an explanation for this.   *(2 marks)*

8   Microbes can live on the surface of the skin.

(a) Give *two* ways in which the body protects itself from these microbes.   *(2 marks)*

(b) Controlling infections in hospitals has become much more difficult in recent years. MRSA is an antibiotic-resistant bacterium.

Explain how the MRSA bacterium has developed resistance to antibiotics.   *(2 marks)*

(c) The pioneer in methods of treating infections in hospitals was Ignaz Semmelweiss. He observed that women whose babies were delivered by doctors in hospital had a death rate of 18% from infections caught in the hospital. Women whose babies were delivered by midwives in the hospital had a death rate of 2%. He observed that doctors often came straight from examining dead bodies to the delivery ward.

In a controlled experiment, Semmelweiss made doctors wash their hands in chloride of lime solution before delivering the babies. The death rate fell to about 2%: down to the same level as the death rate in mothers whose babies were delivered by midwives.

(i) Explain why the death rate fell.   *(1 mark)*

(ii) Explain how Semmelweiss's results could be used to reduce the spread of MRSA in a modern hospital.   *(2 marks)*

13 The immune response

13.1 The immune response

Antibodies

In Chapter 4 you learned that some of the white blood cells can produce **antibodies**. These white blood cells are called **lymphocytes** and they respond when pathogens enter your body. The lymphocytes recognise that the bacteria or viruses are foreign and release the antibodies which stick on the surface of the pathogens.

Antibodies work in two ways. They stick to bacteria to stop them moving around and act as a marker. Other white blood cells, the **phagocytes**, can then recognise them; the phagocytes then **engulf** the bacteria and digest them.

Viruses are much smaller than bacteria and are held in groups so that the phagocytes can target and engulf them more easily.

When lymphocytes produce antibodies in response to an infection we say that you develop **natural immunity**. The lymphocytes will respond very quickly the second time you are infected.

However, there are some diseases which cause very severe symptoms and can be fatal the *first* time you are infected. To protect humans from the consequences of diseases like measles, tuberculosis, polio and, before it was eradicated, smallpox, scientists have developed **vaccines**.

Sitting higher tier

All cells have surface proteins called **antigens** (see page 27). Antigens on foreign cells or pathogens trigger off an immune response. This is why the body rejects donor tissue in transplants; the lymphocytes treat the tissue as if it were a bacteria or virus, producing antibodies to attack the antigens.

Lymphocytes produce specific antibodies. When a pathogen enters the bloodstream the correct type of lymphocyte will be stimulated and it multiples. Eventually sufficient cells are produced to overcome the infection. This takes a few days so you may suffer the symptoms of the disease. However, next time you are infected with the same virus the specific cells respond by releasing antibodies very quickly and you do not become ill. We say that you are **immune** and the specific lymphocytes have an **immunological memory**.

Objectives

How does your immune system work?

What is vaccination?

How are vaccines produced and tested?

What are antigens?

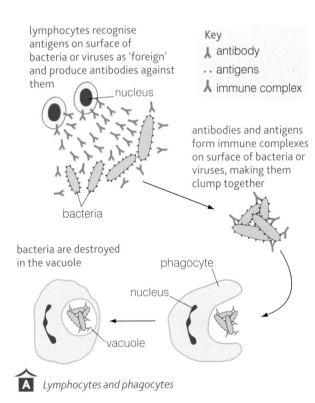

lymphocytes recognise antigens on surface of bacteria or viruses as 'foreign' and produce antibodies against them

nucleus

Key
Λ antibody
.. antigens
Λ immune complex

antibodies and antigens form immune complexes on surface of bacteria or viruses, making them clump together

bacteria

bacteria are destroyed in the vacuole

phagocyte

nucleus

vacuole

A *Lymphocytes and phagocytes*

Vaccines

A vaccine contains a dead or weakened form of the pathogen (usually with the relevant antigen). The following sequence describes what happens following a vaccination which can be by injection or given orally in liquid form:

1   The inactive pathogens enter the bloodstream.
2   Lymphocytes are stimulated.
3   Antibodies are released to destroy the inactive pathogen.
4   The antibodies are gradually lost from the blood but the white cells now have an immunological memory of the shape of the pathogen.
5   Live pathogens enter the body.
6   White blood cells respond very quickly to produce the correct antibodies.
7   Antibodies destroy live pathogens before the person suffers the disease.

This type of immunity is referred to as **artificial immunity** because it results from a vaccine.

Both natural immunity and artificial immunity by vaccination depend on the body producing antibodies quickly during a second infection, so it is **active immunity**.

There may be times when a doctor is confronted with a patient who has a dangerous infection. It may be necessary to inject antibodies. This is called **passive immunity** because the lymphocytes are not involved.

Babies have passive immunity for some diseases because antibodies pass from the mother to the fetus and in the first milk feed after birth.

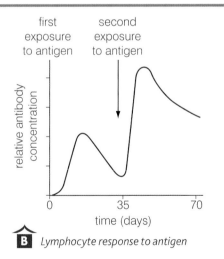

B   *Lymphocyte response to antigen*

The graph shows how the lymphocytes respond to vaccines or pathogens. After the first injection or infection the lymphocytes produce antibodies relatively slowly in the primary response.

Following the second exposure to the same pathogen or vaccination the secondary response is quicker and the concentration of antibodies is greater.

Development of vaccines

At one time, smallpox was a terrible disease which killed about 30% of its victims and left the others deeply scarred by pock marks. In the 10th century, doctors in India and China transferred pus from infected skin into scratches on the skin of healthy people. About 2–3% of those treated died from smallpox, but most were protected from serious illness if they contracted smallpox again. This method of treatment was called 'variolation' and became widely used.

In the 18th century a country doctor, Edward Jenner, observed that milkmaids who had cowpox did not then develop smallpox so he decided to investigate.

Steps in Jenner's research	
Background knowledge	'Variolation' was better than catching smallpox. Cowpox was a mild disease
Observation	Milkmaids who had cowpox did not catch smallpox
Jenner's hypothesis	Something in cowpox protects milkmaids from smallpox
Investigation – Step 1	Took pus from blisters on hand of milkmaid with cowpox and transferred pus to scratch on skin of a healthy boy
Results of Step 1	Boy suffered mild symptoms of cowpox but soon recovered
Investigation – Step 2	Jenner infected boy with pus containing smallpox on two occasions
Results of Step 2	The boy showed no signs of infection on either occasion
Conclusion	The cowpox protected the boy from smallpox
Writing a scientific report	Jenner published his results for the Royal Society – a scientific body
Challenge by other scientists – peer evaluation	Some scientists were not convinced by the first report
Jenner did more tests on other people, including his son. The results were the same and he published them.	His work convinced scientists and he was given research grants to continue his studies

21st century scientists still follow a similar sequence in scientific studies and research in order to get their work accepted.

Modern methods of developing vaccines

When developing new vaccines, the scientists must identify the part of the organism to be used. Vaccines can be prepared from:

- complete pathogens which are killed by heat or chemicals to make them harmless, e.g. whooping cough
- separating parts of the pathogen, e.g. the antigen / protein coat of a virus

Scientists@work

Jenner was made a Fellow of the Royal Society in 1788 for his thorough study on the cuckoo! He used observation, experimentation and dissection to show that the baby cuckoo, not the adult, pushed the eggs of other birds out of their nest.

Did you know ??????

Jenner invented the term 'vaccination' from vacca, the Latin for cow.

- selecting the gene from the pathogen which codes for the protein required and using genetic engineering techniques to produce the protein
- culturing the pathogen and selecting strains which do not cause the disease; this is called weakening or attenuating the virus, e.g. measles and polio.

The vaccine must be tested using tissue culture and animals to show that it stimulates antibody production without damaging the tissue. When safe, the vaccine is tested on large numbers of human volunteers. Once mass vaccination starts, doctors, nurses, and pharmacists are encouraged to report any unusual reactions they notice in individuals. This identifies rare side effects and possible faulty batches of vaccine.

Influenza vaccine is produced by culturing the virus in hens' eggs. Millions of eggs are used every year to prepare sufficient vaccine for winter 'flu epidemics.

Scientists are concerned that it would take too long to produce vaccine doses for everyone who might be affected by a bird flu pandemic, so are looking for new ways to culture the virus.

Did you know ??????

Smallpox was eradicated due to a world-wide vaccination programme and careful tracing of contacts of smallpox sufferers. The World Health Organisation is monitoring the eradication of polio.

Apply what you know

1 Look at the diagram.

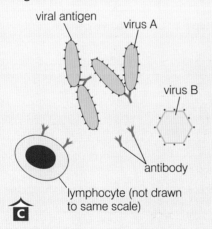

viral antigen
virus A
virus B
antibody
lymphocyte (not drawn to same scale)
C

Explain why the antibodies will only target virus A.

2 Why do we keep getting colds and influenza?

3 What is the advantage of injecting antibodies when treating a dangerous infection, e.g. rabies?

4 What are the differences between the primary and secondary immune responses (see Graph **B**)?

5 How would you evaluate Jenner's work if you were doing a peer evaluation?

6 What is the importance of: **a** testing vaccines with tissues and animals, **b** reporting side effects when the vaccine is in use?

7 Can you suggest why hens' eggs would not be suitable for producing vaccine for preventing a bird flu epidemic in humans?

Foul facts

In the 20th century smallpox killed 300 million people, one-third of those infected. The Spanish conquered the Aztecs and Incas in the 16th century, when many of the latter died from smallpox due to lack of immunity.

14 Cancer

14.1 Cancer

What is a tumour?

In the previous chapters you learned that cells divide by mitosis to enable growth and repair of the body tissues. This process is normally well controlled but occasionally a cell can change due to several mutations of its genes and it will divide in an uncontrolled way. This abnormal growth forms a group of cells called a **tumour**. If the tumour is enclosed and stays in one place it is called **benign** and is only a problem if it compresses other tissue, e.g. in the brain. Treatment for benign tumours may include surgery to remove the tumour or use of drugs or radiation to shrink and possibly destroy it.

Malignant tumours are those which can spread to healthy tissue and are the ones we call **cancer**.

Objectives

What is cancer?

What causes cancer?

How is cancer diagnosed and treated?

How was smoking linked to lung cancer?

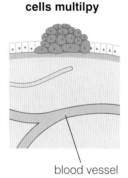

normal cells **abnormal cells** **abnormal cells multilpy** **malignant or invasive cancer**

primary cancer

boundary

local invasion

angiogenesis: tumours grow their own blood vessels

metastasis: cells move away from primary tumour and invade other parts of the body via blood vessels and lymph vessels

lymph vessel

blood vessel

 A *How a malignant tumour starts and spreads*

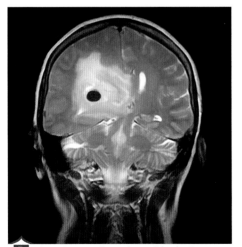

B *An MRI scan of a patient with a brain tumour*

Scientists@work

Many health professionals are involved in the diagnosis and treatment of cancer. Other scientists, including geneticists, dieticians and environmental scientists, carry out research into the causes of cancer.

The lymph system

The lymph system has vessels similar to blood vessels but it carries a clear liquid and white blood cells, called **lymph**, between the tissues and the blood system. Lymph passes through lymph glands and may transport cancer cells to these regions. If the immune system is unable to destroy the cancer cells then a **secondary** tumour may grow. This is why lymph glands close to a tumour are often removed in case cancer cells have spread to them. Secondary tumours also occur in other parts of the body.

There are over 200 different forms of cancer, affecting different tissues in the body. The most common cause of cancer deaths is lung cancer; prostate, breast and bowel cancers are also very common.

What causes cancer?

There are many causes of cancer including **carcinogens** (cancer-causing chemicals), environmental factors such as **ultraviolet light** (radiation from the Sun) and X-rays, diet, our age, genes and viruses. Several of these may cause a particular person's cancer.

C *Some common cancers and possible risk factors; remember that individuals may get cancer for a range of reasons*

Site of cancer	Probable cause / risk
Lung cancer	Carcinogens in cigarette smoke – 95% of lung cancers
	Other carcinogens, e.g. asbestos
Breast cancer	Very complex , but includes long-term exposure to oestrogen, high fat levels in older women, genes
Prostate cancer	Age, overweight, high fat diet, family members with breast cancer, ethnic group
Mouth, tongue, oesophagus	Smoking and drinking alcohol
Cervical cancer	Human papilloma virus (HPV)
Skin cancer	Ultraviolet light from Sun / sun beds
Bowel cancer	Age – over 80% are 60+, low fibre diet

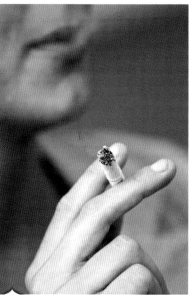

D *The carcinogens in cigarette smoke can cause lung and other cancers*

Diagnosing cancer

If a person has an unusual lump, bleeding from the bowel, changes in moles or other worries, a GP may refer him or her to an oncologist for further tests. These will include blood tests, X-rays and other scans to look inside the body, and possibly a biopsy where a small piece of tissue is cut out and examined by a pathologist.

Treatments for cancer

Nowadays there are many treatment options for curing or slowing the progress of a cancer:

- surgery to remove the tumour
- chemotherapy, which uses drugs to kill cancer cells
- radiotherapy, which uses high energy rays to kill cancer cells
- both chemotherapy and radiotherapy may be used to shrink tumours before surgery
- bone marrow or stem cell therapy may be used to replace cells in the bone marrow which have been killed with the cancer cells.

How are links made between cancer and its causes?

Much cancer research about causes involves asking people, with cancer, questions about their lifestyle and family history and looking for common answers. In 1951, a doctor working for the Medical Research Council, Richard Doll, published a paper suggesting that lung cancer is caused by smoking as a result of surveying 700 patients. Some people, especially cigarette manufacturers, were sceptical, so he looked for more proof. Doll's research team asked over 40 000 doctors if they smoked and then monitored their health. All the doctors who developed lung cancer over the next few years were smokers. The link had been made. In Doll's study the doctors who did not smoke acted as the control group for comparison.

Later studies have validated these results, as other scientists repeated the investigations and confirmed them. It has been shown that cigarette smoke contains many chemicals which are carcinogenic and may affect non-smokers. This is why governments have banned smoking in public places.

Time will tell if the numbers of cancer and other lung disorders reduces in both smokers and non-smokers as a result.

Did you know ??????

Richard Doll gave up smoking in his 40s because he was so convinced by the evidence. He died in 2005 aged 92.

Did you know ??????

New treatments for cancer include biological therapy, hormone therapy and gene therapy.

Prevention is better than cure

The media are always telling us about 'superfoods' which may help to prevent cancer, but most of these reports refer to small scale studies and need confirmation by more rigorous research.

In 2008 widespread use of a vaccine, to protect girls against the human papilloma virus, was introduced in the UK. This should significantly reduce the incidence of cervical cancer.

Reducing fat and red meat, increasing fresh foods containing fibre, and covering up in bright sunlight may help to protect against some cancers. But the single, most effective, way to reduce risk is not to start smoking or to stop immediately if you are a smoker.

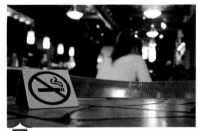

E *Smoking in public places was banned in England in 2007*

Find out ... O⸚

Use some of the following organisations' websites to find out more about cancer:

- Cancer Research UK
- Cancer Help
- NHS Direct
- BUPA

AQA *Examiner's tip*

- Always give a scientific reason when asked to 'explain'.
- Make sure you understand the limitations of an investigation.
- Look for trends when describing graphs.
- Do *not* assume that all research is biased but *do* identify the source of the data – is it from patients, relatives, the media or scientists?

Foul facts

Worldwide 15 billion cigarettes are sold daily – 10 million per minute.

80 000–100 000 children start smoking every day, about half in Asia.

Every 8 seconds someone dies from tobacco use.

1 in 3 cigarettes is smoked in China. If this continues, 80 million Chinese will die of lung cancer in the next 25 years.

In the UK 29% of *all* cancer deaths are caused by smoking.

Did you know ??????

In 1948, 82% of UK men smoked; in 2002 this had dropped to 30%.

Apply what you know

1. What advice would you give to a 14-year-old girl to help reduce her risk of developing cancer?

2. Why is it important to include control groups in surveys and other investigations?

3. 5–10% of people with lung cancer are non-smokers. Does this invalidate Doll's research findings?

4. In some cases, oncologists are not keen to perform surgery on a tumour. Can you suggest why?

5. Look at Graph **F** suggesting links between smoking and cancer. What can you deduce from the graph?

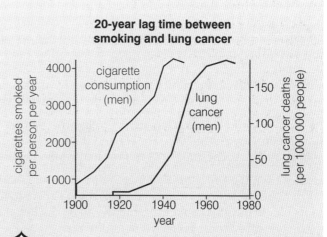

F *The trends in these graphs suggest a link between smoking and cancer*

15 Twenty-first century health

15.1 Twenty-first century health

In the middle of the 20th century people were very afraid of being told they had cancer because the death rate was very high. Treatments were often experimental and little was known about some of the causes. Medical research focussed on 'finding a cure for cancer'. As scientists learned more about human genes and the range of causes for different cancers, they realised there would not be a single cure. Nowadays many types of cancer are treatable with new drugs. Modern scanning equipment, and screening techniques, often detect cancer at early stages in the development of the disease. However the cost of developing and testing cancer drugs is very high. This also applies to treatments for many other serious diseases and doctors often have to face difficult decisions about who should be offered new drugs or procedures such as transplants.

Objectives

Who is responsible for our health?

What are the modern health problems?

What are the constraints on health professionals?

Are alternative therapies of any value?

Ethics and economics

Sometimes doctors will insist that a person changes their lifestyle before they are offered medical treatment. It can be dangerous for an obese person to have an operation, and IVF is less successful with obese women, so they may be advised to lose weight first. In other situations a surgeon may tell a smoker to stop smoking for several months before an operation. A heavy drinker might be asked to stop drinking alcohol while waiting for a liver transplant. There are medical, economic and ethical reasons for this advice. It costs a lot of money to give someone an organ transplant, donors are rare and there are many people on the waiting list. Doctors need to be sure that the patient has the best chance of a full recovery.

Life expectancy

Now that we have new drugs for treatment and prevention of disease, and techniques such as keyhole surgery which enable people to recover quickly, our prospects of reaching a healthy old age are improving. But increasing numbers of elderly people can bring a range of new demands and higher health costs. Care home places are required for patients with dementia, or for those disabled by strokes, and people with limited mobility may need support in their own homes.

In 1981 65 year-old men could expect to live for another 13 years; this rose to 17 years in 2005. For women the figures are 17 years and almost 20 years. The gap between men and women has narrowed.

Figures from the Office for National Statistics (ONS) show that boys born in the UK between 2005 and 2007 could expect to live to 77.2 years old, while girls could expect to live to 81.5. How might changes in lifestyle affect these projected mortality rates?

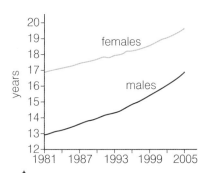

A Life expectancy for 65 year-olds in the UK; you can see that both men and women now live longer than in 1981 and the trend is upwards

Eating habits

B *Data from a health survey for England to illustrate the change in overweight and obesity levels in children aged 2–15 between 1995 and 2004*

Gender	Age (years)	Percentage overweight in 1995	Percentage obese in 1995	Percentage overweight including obese in 1995	Percentage overweight in 2004	Percentage obese in 2004	Percentage overweight including obese in 2004
Boys	2–10	12.9	9.6	22.5	14.6	15.9	30.5
Boys	11–15	13.4	13.5	26.9	12.8	24.2	37.0
Boys	2–15	13.1	10.9	24.0	13.9	19.2	33.1
Girls	2–10	12.6	10.3	22.9	14.8	12.8	27.6
Girls	11–15	13.9	15.4	29.3	19.3	26.7	46.0
Girls	2–15	13.1	12.0	25.0	16.6	18.5	35.1

Dieticians and nutritionists have been warning other health professionals, the government and parents that there is danger of an obesity 'epidemic' in the UK. The figures in the table confirm that about a third of children are either overweight or obese, an increase of about 10% in 10 years. These children are more likely to suffer from heart disease, type 2 diabetes, or both, at a much younger age which could reduce their life expectancy.

Exercise habits

Compared with 100 years ago, many of us are walking less and much of our leisure time is spent sitting at a computer or watching the television. Consequently we use less energy and increase our risk of obesity and heart disease.

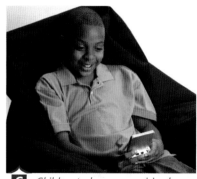

C *Children today are exercising less*

Drinking habits

Recent surveys show that the number of teenagers who start drinking alcohol at a young age is going down, but those that do drink are consuming a higher number of units. The long term effects of this consumption are not yet known, but it is known that alcohol can alter the functioning of the brain and adolescence is a critical stage in brain development.

Health reports suggest that about two-thirds of the English population drink alcohol at least once a week. A significant number of these drink more than the recommended daily amounts (of 2 units for women and 3 for men) at least twice a week. Heavy drinking is particularly dangerous in the case of pregnant women.

Embryos can be affected by alcohol which crosses the placenta. In severe cases the child can be born with **fetal alcohol syndrome**, which may include learning difficulties, hyperactivity and attention problems.

Drinking alcohol not only damages the brain but can also increase the risk of obesity, cancer, alcoholic liver disease and heart disease in regular drinkers.

Over-the-counter drug habits

Of the £11 billion spent in the UK on medication, about £2 billion is spent by the public for **over-the-counter** (OTC) pills, creams and liquid preparations to treat headaches, skin conditions, coughs, colds and a wide range of other minor ailments. Some OTC drugs can be found on general sale, while others can only be sold at a registered pharmacy so that pharmacists have some control over who buys them.

Recently a low dose **statin** was released to be sold as OTC. Statins reduce blood cholesterol levels and consequently the risk of cardiovascular disease. Pharmacists offer health advice and cholesterol tests to ensure that people at moderate risk of heart disease are targeted correctly. Patients at high risk are diagnosed by doctors and prescribed higher dose statins which are dispensed by pharmacists but not sold directly to the public.

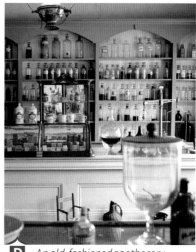

D An old-fashioned apothecary

Alternative therapies

Some people prefer not to take drugs to treat headaches, backpain and symptoms such as nausea. In fact long term use of some painkillers can lead to addiction and a reduction in effectiveness. There are a large number of therapies which are referred to as '**alternative**' and some of them are recommended by doctors to complement orthodox treatment.

Mind therapies include relaxation techniques, hypnotherapy, meditation and art therapy. They help people to feel better by reducing the symptoms or emotional distress caused by serious illness. Psychoprophylaxis is a relaxation technique taught to pregnant women to help them control the pain of labour.

Acupuncture, which originated in China, has been used for about 4000 years. The philosophy of acupuncture is that human health is the result of harmony among bodily functions (physiology) and between the body and nature. Disease occurs when this harmony is disrupted, so acupuncture is used to restore the state of harmony. Treatments involve inserting steel needles into a few (usually 4–10) of the 365 acupuncture points in the body, depending on the condition being treated. Many people have benefited from acupuncture treatment, particularly as a method of pain relief.

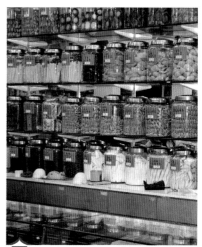

E Chinese herbal medicines

Clinical trials have shown that acupuncture can help some conditions such as post-operative nausea, but it is very difficult to test the therapy. Trials should involve placebos; designing 'sham' acupuncture for comparison is clearly a problem.

Alternative chemical therapies include **homeopathy** and **herbal** medicine.

The principle of homeopathy is that if large doses of a chemical cause a symptom, then minute doses will cure it. Very dilute solutions of toxic substances are administered which do little harm and some patients find beneficial.

Many medicines are derived from plants. Aspirin is derived from willow bark, and morphine is derived from opium poppies. Pharmacists test newly discovered plants for possible healing properties in the hope of extracting a single chemical. Herbalists tend to use unpurified extracts

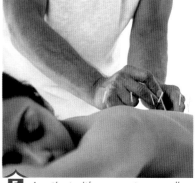

F A patient with acupuncture needles inserted

from the whole plant or combine different herbs together. This means that the various chemical components can be in different proportions which make clinical testing less reliable.

As more people turn to alternative therapies they should be made aware that some can actually interfere with drugs from a doctor, e.g. a patient taking **warfarin** to reduce blood clotting should not take **ginseng** because it alters the clotting time. Other herbs may interfere with antibiotics or the contraceptive pill, making them less effective.

One of the problems for the public is knowing who to believe. Hearsay or anecdotal evidence is often used to promote alternative therapies, so it is important to balance this with scientific evidence from health professionals.

Apply what you know

Unlike diseases caused by pathogens, disorders resulting from overeating, lack of exercise and drinking alcohol are preventable but they have an enormous impact on the National Health Service in the UK.

Use your knowledge from previous chapters and the information above, to answer the questions.

1 What advice would you give to a group of teenagers to prevent them becoming obese and developing diabetes or heart disease later in life? Draw up a list of 'dos' and 'don'ts'.

2 Imagine that you are responsible for deciding which of two patients should be given a heart transplant. What factors might you have to take into consideration?

3 Make lists of the reasons for and against drinking alcohol.

4 Who is responsible for our health? A mother took her 10 year-old son to the doctor because he was sleeping badly. The doctor suggested the boy was very overweight. Instead of prescribing sleeping pills he referred the boy to a dietician.

Make a table using the following headings and suggest how each is responsible for the health of the woman's son. Try to think of two suggestions for each column

The son	His parents	The doctor	The government	The food industry

5 Garlic is believed to have cholesterol lowering properties. How would you design a trial to find out if garlic works as well as statins?

Did you know ??????

In 2004, the UK government estimated that alcohol misuse costs the health service between £1.4 and £1.7 billion per year.

Find out ...

Use the internet to find out more about acupuncture, homeopathy and herbal medicine.

Foul facts

A herbal treatment for osteoarthritis contains turmeric, devil's claw, ginseng, white willow, liquorice and oats.

AQA Examiner's tip

Evaluate health-related articles in a scientific way:

- Is the information reliable?
- Is it factual or hearsay?
- Was it written by an expert or a journalist?
- Is scientific evidence quoted?
- Is the article balanced?
- What are the pros and cons?

There are two parts to the controlled assessment, which forms 25% of the Human Health and Physiology qualification:

- the **Practical Skills Assessment** (PSA) worth 6 marks
- the **Investigative Skills Assignment** (ISA) worth 34 marks.

The **PSA** will be assessed during normal practical lessons. To gain maximum marks you should be able to:

- Conduct your practical work in a safe and well organised manner.
- Demonstrate competence with a range of equipment, some of which is quite complex, e.g. using colour standards such as litmus paper is relatively straightforward, but a colorimeter is more complex and gives more accurate, quantitative data.
- Take all measurements to an appropriate level of accuracy, e.g. if all the volumes lie between the markings on a measuring cylinder you would need a graduated pipette or burette to give accurate readings.
- Present, while the work is in progress, the data collected in a suitable table.

The **ISA** is started as class practical work and ends with a written paper which is completed in lesson time under test conditions. The test questions will examine your understanding of the particular practical you have done and your knowledge and understanding of How Science Works. There are two sections in the test:

- **Section 1** concentrates entirely on the method and results of your own practical.
- **Section 2** includes data from a new, but similar, situation and will test your ability to apply what you did in class to this new scenario.

AQA supply two ISAs per year for Human Health and Physiology. You may perform one or both but you cannot repeat them. All work is supervised by your teacher and there is no coursework to do at home.

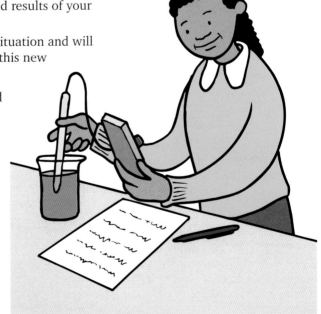

Example of PSA work

On page 18 there is a description of how to test foods for energy content. It involves:

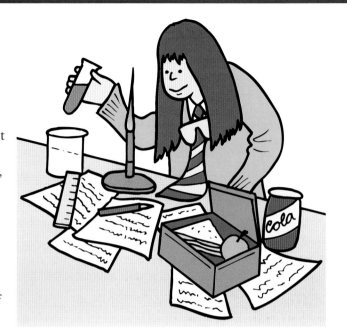

▧ Working safely – using the Bunsen burner.

▧ Being organised – transferring the food from flame to test tube quickly involves deciding where the equipment will stand, and don't forget the flame must not heat the water.

▧ Accurate measurements – volume of water used, mass of food, temperature of water.

Example of ISA work

The topic for an ISA could relate to work on enzymes.

For example, you could investigate the effect of temperature on amylase activity on the digestion of starch.

Before starting the investigation you need to be clear what is likely to happen by asking questions such as:

▧ What will I change?

▧ How can I measure activity?

These will allow you to collect valid data.

Before starting, you should complete the following check list:

▧ What is the independent variable? [temperature]

▧ What type of variable is this? [continuous]

▧ What is the dependent variable? [the time it takes for the starch to disappear]

▧ How can I make sure it is a fair test? [keep everything the same except temperature]

▧ What are the control variables? [concentration and volume of solutions used]

▧ What range shall I use for the independent variable? [0°C–100°C, 20°C–70°C or 15°C–45°C?]

▧ What intervals should I choose? [every 5°C, 10°C, or 20°C?]

▧ How can I measure time more precisely? [use a stopwatch rather than a wall clock]

▧ How can I make my results more reliable? [repetitions of the tests at each temperature]

▧ What headings do I need on my table? [Temperature (°C), Time (minutes or seconds?) Is minutes or seconds more precise and therefore nearer to the true value – more accurate?]

▧ What type of graph should I use to present data? [a line graph]

When evaluating the results you need to look for anomalies, describe the relationship between the dependent and independent variables and decide if you used the best range or intervals or did sufficient repeats to give reliable results.

Chapters 13–16

1   (a)   Choose from the words below to copy and complete the sentences about curing diseases:

antibiotics   antibodies   anti-toxins   painkillers   statins

The substances made by white blood cells to kill pathogens are called …

The substances made by white blood cells to counteract poisons produced by pathogens are called …

Medicines which kill bacteria are called …   *(3 marks)*

(b)   **Table 1** shows some statements which may be related to active immunity, to passive immunity or to both. Copy the table, then complete it by placing a tick in the box if the statement is true or a cross in the box if the statement is not true.

Table 1

Statement	Active immunity	Passive immunity
Antibodies are produced if the body is re-infected by the same pathogen		
An antibody reacts with an antigen		
Antibodies are received in breast milk		
Weakened microorganisms are used in the vaccine		

(4 marks)

(c)   Health visitors advise parents to have their children immunised with the MMR vaccine. The MMR vaccine protects children from measles, mumps and rubella. All vaccinations involve some risk.

Table 2 shows the risk of developing harmful effects:

from the disease if a child is *not* given the MMR vaccine

if a child *is* given the MMR vaccine.

Table 2

Harmful effect	Risk of getting the harmful effect from the disease (if not vaccinated)	Risk of getting the harmful effect from MMR vaccine
Convulsions	1 in 200	1 in 1000
Meningitis	1 in 3000	Less than 1 in 1 000 000
Brain damage	1 in 8000	0

A mother is considering if she should have her child vaccinated with the MMR vaccine.

Use information from the table to persuade the mother that she should have her child vaccinated.   *(3 marks)*

2 Antibodies help to defend the body against disease.

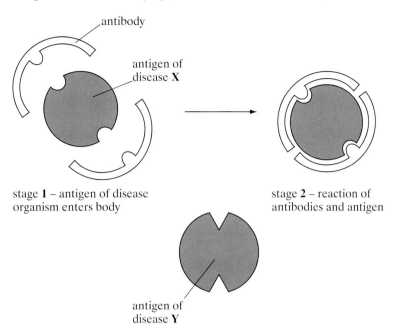

(a) The diagram represents the reaction of antibody and antigen for disease **X.**

Using the diagram to help you, suggest why the body's defence against disease **X** would not be effective against disease **Y.** *(2 marks)*

(b) Tuberculosis is a disease which is caused by a bacterium. The body is able to produce antibodies to destroy the bacteria which cause the disease. Some people are naturally immune. A person can be tested to find if they are immune. Use information from the diagrams to help you answer the questions.

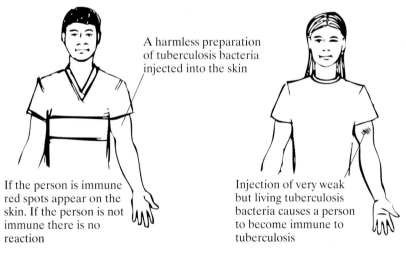

(i) Suggest the possible cause of the reaction when a person who is already immune is tested, as shown in diagram **A.** *(1 mark)*

(ii) Explain why the injection of tuberculosis bacteria (diagram **B**) causes immunity but does not cause the disease. *(3 marks)*

3 Immunologists have developed a vaccine against malaria. A trial of this vaccine was carried out in South America. **Table 3** shows some more data collected during this trial. It shows the total number and percentage of people in different age groups who caught malaria during the first year of the trial.

Table 3

Age group	Vaccinated group		Control group	
(years)	Total number	Percentage	Total number	Percentage
1–4	3	0.07	13	0.32
5–9	32	0.44	43	0.58
10–14	36	0.57	58	0.75
15–44	68	0.62	83	0.57

(a) (i) Explain why it was necessary to have a control group. *(1 mark)*

   (ii) How would the treatment of the control group differ from the vaccinated group? *(1 mark)*

(b) Explain the reason for giving the percentage of people who caught malaria as well as the total number. *(2 marks)*

(c) The researchers concluded that the vaccine was most effective with people 1–4 years old.

   Does the data from the table support this conclusion? Give the reason for your answer *(1 mark)*

(d) Give *three* ethical issues that researchers should consider when conducting a trial such as this.

   (3 marks)

4 Cancer is still a major cause of death in the UK.

(a) Some tumours are benign and some are malignant.

   (i) Give *one* way in which a benign tumour differs from a malignant tumour. *(1 mark)*

   (ii) Describe *two* ways in which a tumour may cause harm to the body. *(2 marks)*

(b) Oncologists advise patients on the risk factors for cancer.

   (i) Explain the link between sunbathing and skin cancer. *(2 marks)*

   (ii) Suggest why fair-skinned people are at a greater risk of skin cancer than dark-skinned people when sunbathing. *(1 mark)*

   (iii) Suggest why people with a family history of cancer are at a greater risk of cancer than those with no family history of cancer. *(2 marks)*

5 Doctors advise all men over the age of 50 to have regular checks for prostate cancer. The most common test is the PSA test.

An antigen called PSA is present in the blood of men in the early stages of prostate cancer. There is a blood test for PSA. The test uses antibodies to PSA. The stages in the test are shown in the diagram on the next page.

(a) What is an antigen? *(2 marks)*

(b) (i) Explain why this test detects prostate cancer, but not any other disease. *(2 marks)*

   (ii) Explain why there will not be a colour change if the blood sample does not contain PSA. *(2 marks)*

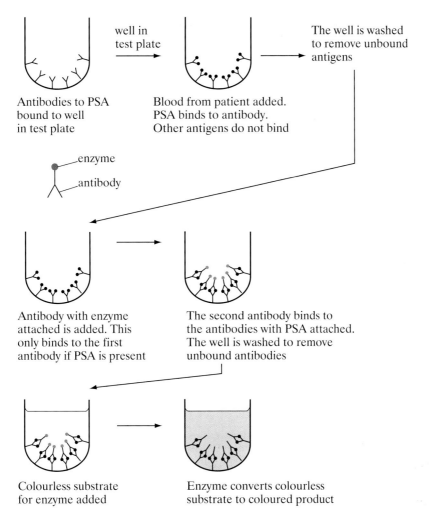

well in test plate

Antibodies to PSA bound to well in test plate

Blood from patient added. PSA binds to antibody. Other antigens do not bind

The well is washed to remove unbound antigens

enzyme

antibody

Antibody with enzyme attached is added. This only binds to the first antibody if PSA is present

The second antibody binds to the antibodies with PSA attached. The well is washed to remove unbound antibodies

Colourless substrate for enzyme added

Enzyme converts colourless substrate to coloured product

(c) Read the passage.

The PSA test along with a digital rectal exam (DRE) helps detect prostate cancer in men age 50 and older. During a DRE, a doctor inserts a gloved finger into the rectum and feels the prostate gland through the rectal wall to check for bumps or abnormal areas. Doctors often use the PSA test and DRE as prostate cancer screening tests; together, these tests can help doctors detect prostate cancer in men who have no symptoms of the disease.

It is not clear if the benefits of PSA screening outweigh the risks of follow-up diagnostic tests and cancer treatments. For example, the PSA test may detect small cancers that would never become life threatening. This situation, called overdiagnosis, puts men at risk for complications from unnecessary treatment such as surgery or radiation.

Should all men over 50 be screened for prostate cancer?

Explain the reasons for your answer.

6   Colon cancer is sometimes known as the 'silent killer'.

One hypothesis for the cause of cancer of the colon (large intestine) is that *Clostridium* bacteria present in the gut can convert bile steroids into cancer-causing substances. The concentrations of bile steroids and numbers of *Clostridium* bacteria were measured in people with colon cancer and in controls without colon cancer. **Table 4** shows the results.

Table 4

Concentration of bile steroids	Number of *Clostridium* bacteria	Percentage of cancer patients	Percentage of controls
High	High	76	9
High	Low	13	8
Low	High	7	34
Low	Low	4	49

(a) Do the results support the hypothesis that *Clostridium* bacteria convert bile steroids into substances which cause colon cancer?

Explain the reasons for your answer.   *(2 marks)*

(b) The results indicate that other factors may be involved in causing colon cancer. Explain how.   *(1 mark)*

(c) Bacteria are once again being used in the war on cancer. Scientists have genetically engineered a harmless strain of *Clostridium* to carry the gene for an enzyme. This enzyme converts a harmless 'prodrug' into an active drug which acts as a powerful toxin. In people, this strain of *Clostridium* will only grow in tumours. Scientists hope that when they inject the prodrug into a cancer patient's blood, the bacteria willconvert it into an active drug. This will destroy tumours from the inside, leaving healthy tissues unharmed.

Explain how the use of antibodies results in a drug only killing cancer cells.   *(2 marks)*

7   Scientists study the effect of smoking on the number of people dying from lung cancer. **Graph 1** shows the number of people who died from lung cancer in this country between 1950 and 2000.

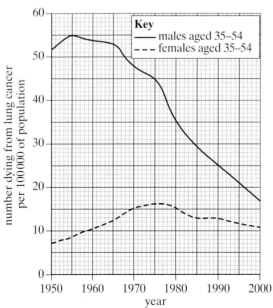

(a) Describe how the number of men who died from lung cancer changed between 1960 and 2000.   *(2 marks)*

(b) Describe *two* differences between the numbers of men and women who died from lung cancer between 1960 and 2000.   *(2 marks)*

(c)   A town in this country had 500 000 inhabitants in 1955. How many men aged 35–54 from that town are likely to have died from lung cancer in 1955?   *(1 mark)*

(d)   **Graph 2** shows the percentage of the population who smoked between 1950 and 2000.

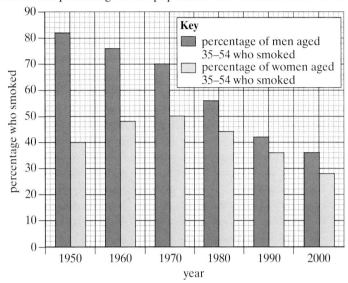

Explain how the data from Graphs 1 and 2 support the hypothesis that smoking increases the risk of getting lung cancer.   *(2 marks)*

8   Epidemiologists compile statistics on risk factors for diseases. The graph shows male alcohol-related death rates by age group in the UK between 1991 and 2006.

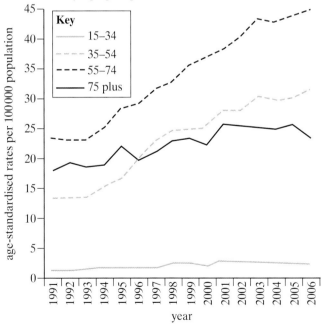

(a)   (i)   Describe the trend in alcohol-related deaths in 55–74 year-olds.   *(2 marks)*

       (ii)   55–74 year-olds always had the most alcohol-related deaths.
               Suggest an explanation for this.   *(2 marks)*

(b)   Suggest an explanation for the increase in the number of alcohol-related deaths in 35–54 year-old men.   *(2 marks)*

(c)   Doctors are concerned about the increase in binge-drinking in 15–34 year-olds.
       Suggest an explanation for their concern.   *(2 marks)*

Answers to 'Apply what you know'

1 Cells and cell processes

1.1 Cell structure and organisation

1 Egg cell, sperm cell, red blood cell, nerve cell, muscle cell

2 Egg cell and sperm cell for reproduction; red blood cell to transport oxygen; nerve cell to coordinate the sense around the body / transport electrical impulses / allow us to feel things [or any other good explanation]; muscle cell for movement

3 Red blood cell, (the blood, the heart, the circulation system) nerve cell, (nerve tissues, the nervous system), muscle cell (muscle tissues, the muscle system)

4 Advantage: instant energy when needed; disadvantage: limited amount of energy released / production of lactic acid which causes muscle fatigue and cramp

5 Muscle cells and sperm cells

6 Oxygen, glucose and other nutrients, e.g. amino acids. Explanation: oxygen and glucose are needed for aerobic respiration, nutrients are used for cell growth and to make new cells, e.g. amino acids are built into proteins

1.2 Cell Processes

1 An enzyme

2 Glucose dissolves in water and changes the concentration of the cytoplasm. This would cause water to enter the cell by osmosis. Glycogen will *not* draw water into the cell, and will *not* diffuse out of the cell because it is insoluble.

3 Muscle and sperm cells need a lot of energy for movement.

4 An enzyme

2 Nutrition

2.1 Nutrition

1 [Own answer]

2 Movement, chemical reactions, warming the body, repairing cells

3 They are growing and should be very active.

4 The growing embryo requires a lot of energy.

5

a Reduce the fat content. Poach the egg, grill the bacon and sausage and toast the bread (no butter!)

b It will have less fat and more vitamins and minerals.

c The plate with more vegetables

6 Vitamin C

7 Decreased wound healing, decreased ability to fight infection

2.2 Food labelling and food testing

1

a Barry's Best Beans

b Harry's Healthy Beans

c Sally's Salmon

d Barry's Best Beans

e Sally's Salmon

f Harry's Healthy Beans – less salt, less sugar but has slightly more fat than Barry's Best

3 Digestion

3.1 Physical and chemical breakdown of food

1 Acid in the fruit softens the enamel. Brushing removes the enamel with the food.

2 The nerve endings have been exposed, which are pain receptors.

3.2 The human digestive system

1 No, glucose is soluble and small enough to pass through cell surface membranes.

2 Enzyme: amylase; substrate: starch; product: reducing sugar; independent variable: presence of active amylase; dependent variable: presence of sugar; control variables: temperature, time

3 Cystic fibrosis: the pancreatic enzymes cannot be secreted onto the food in the small intestine and nutrients cannot diffuse through the sticky mucus covering the villi. Coeliac disease: the surface area for absorption is reduced.

4 Blood and the ciculation system

4.1 Blood

1 Water; cells; plasma; soluble food, e.g. glucose, amino acids; gases, e.g. oxygen, carbon dioxide; hormones; proteins for clotting; waste materials, e.g. urea

2 There is more room for the haemoglobin. The surface area to volume ratio of the cell is increased for more rapid diffusion of oxygen.

3 The clots would block the blood capillaries and prevent materials reaching the cells.

4 Mix sample with known blood types, look for clumping. If suspects had a different blood type from that found, they were likely to be innocent. But so many people have the same blood group a suspect could argue it was not his.

4.2 Circulation

1 It keeps the blood flowing round the body and supplies oxygen and food to cells.

2 To stop smoking, reduce alcohol consumption, change diet, increase exercise. Reduce the risk factors of high blood pressure, high blood cholesterol, diabetes, obesity.

3 Reduce saturated fat intake, reduce salt and sugar intake, increase fresh fruit and vegetables in the diet.

4 More activity increases the need for oxygen to the muscles. The heart rate increases to increase the supply of oxygenated blood.

5

a e.g. dangerous, not done before, patient very ill, should doctors do this? Is it interfering with nature?

b e.g. economic – transplants are very expensive but balanced by cost of other treatment, lack of donors, stem cell research is costly and highly complex – difficult to grow an organ from groups of cells

6 You will need to consider information about the costs of various methods, health of patient, time of recovery, use of stem cell technology, should smokers/obese people/ alcoholics be treated, the need for immunosuppressant drugs plus any suggestions specific to a new method.

5 Gas exchange

5.1 Gas exchange

1 The intercostal muscles relax, the diaphragm relaxes, the rib cage falls, the internal pressure goes up, the volume goes down.

2 To keep the airways open

3 There is a high concentration of oxygen in the air compared with the blood. There is a high concentration of carbon dioxide in the blood compared with the air.

4 Large surface area to volume ratio, close to network of blood capillaries, very thin wall

5 The surface area of the alveoli is reduced, less gas exchange takes place, less oxygen reaches the cells, less respiration means less energy.

6 You breathe deeper and more often.

7

a One tube for blood in, the other for blood out

b Bacteria and dust will be removed by filtering. Oxygen from the air will diffuse across to the blood, carbon dioxide will diffuse out.

c Blood clots could block the patient's blood vessels and cause a heart attack or stroke.

d i The portable device means they are not restricted to a hospital bed.

ii An internal device would allow the patient to walk about and do normal activities. It may mean they do not need a lung transplant.

e Cost, finding suitable materials, making the device small enough to fit in the chest

6 Gas exchange

6.1 Excretion

1

a Less water is lost due to sweating, so more water is lost in the urine.

b More water is lost in the sweat, so the kidneys reabsorb more water and less is lost in the urine; eventually you could become dehydrated.

2

a Diffusion

b Osmosis

3 Alcohol shows in urine 1.5–2 hours after consumption, so will not show the current blood alcohol concentration. The concentration of urine varies depending on a person's level of hydration and their metabolic rate.

4 [Students need to use the tables to compare cost, convenience for patient, risk from infection, availability of dialysis machines and donors, dietary restrictions.]

5 Dialysis costs = £189 million; drug costs = £30 million

The government can:

Promote the need for donors with advertising campaigns. Bring in legislation for an 'opting-out system': people register to say they do not want to be donors rather than carry donor cards.
Ethical issues might include:
People believe they won't be kept alive after an accident if their organs are needed.
Some people have religious objections to giving blood and organs.
Doctors must decide on medical grounds, but may be influenced by who is 'more deserving' e.g. a young patient versus old, a non-smoker versus a smoker.

7 Nervous systems, hormones and coordination

7.1 Nervous system

1 Voluntary: pick up cake; reflex: other three.

2 Protects from: burning skin, damage to retina, choking by blocked windpipe.

7.2 The eye

1 Clouding of the lens (cataract), damage to cornea, damage to retina caused by injury or diabetes, damage to optic nerve.

7.3 Hormones and coordination

1 Control by the endocrine system is slower, may target a wider area and the effects last longer.

2 Nervous system – blinking, flinching, sneezing, focusing, swatting a fly

Endocrine system – blood sugar, growing, menstrual cycle, metabolic rate

3 Pros: Without the dog experiments insulin would not have been discovered. Diabetics would have died if the pig insulin was not made available.

Cons: Some people object to using animals believing it is cruel. Many pigs were needed. Some patients were allergic to pig insulin. There are more diabetics now: genetically engineered insulin can be made quickly and does not involve animals. Human insulin will not be rejected. Some people object to putting human genes in bacteria.

4 More oxygen and glucose will reach the muscles for aerobic respiration, more energy released for running etc.

5 The blood water increases – detected – ADH not produced – less water absorbed by kidney – decrease in water content in blood.

6 There is still some ADH in the bloodstream.

7.4 Homeostasis

1 Cells would lose water by osmosis and shrink.

2 Less sweating when colder so more water lost in urine

3 The layer of dead skin cells is thicker / there are fewer heat receptors.

4 The fabric prevents radiation from the skin.

5 The core temperature rises, sweating increases. If too much water is lost the core temperature continues to rise to dangerous levels. Drinks rehydrate the body.

6 If the core body temperature continues to fall, enzyme action slows to dangerous levels.

7 To maintain aerobic respiration and energy release

8 The activity increases the rate of heat loss and increases exhaustion.

8 Muscles, bones and movement

8.1 Bones, muscles and joints

1
a Brain, by the cranium, but also eyes and ears, etc.
b Heart and lungs
c Spinal cord

2
a Cervical
b Thoracic
c Lumbar

8.2 Skeletal health

1 More friction between bones due to loss of cartilage

2 The mineral salts would dissolve.

3 Excess weight can cause strain on the back and gives the knees more weight to support. Calcium is needed to strengthen bones. The heavy bag is causing her to bend to one side, pulling the vertebral column out of line. Light exercise will help to lose weight, and strengthen the muscles and other tissues around joints but won't aggravate the possible cartilage damage to her knees. The physiotherapist can advise on the correct exercise, assess and treat the injuries to her joints and advise her about posture and diet.

4
a The spaces between the bone tissue are bigger and the bone tissue is thineer in the osteoporotic bone
b The bone has lost strength and the thinner patches are more likely to snap.

9 Human reproduction and birth

9.1 Human reproduction

1 Eggs and sperm will not multiply into new cells.

2 Mitosis

3 The embryo is prevented from developing into a human.

4 The cells contain the woman's chromosomes / match the woman's body cells / will not be rejected.

5 Organs contain many tissues which have to be organised in exactly the correct positions.

9.2 Fertilisation and birth

1 The blood groups may be different; the mother's blood pressure would be higher; there would be no barrier.

2 Fetus needs a whole range of nutrients (see 2.1).

3 If mother uses up carbohydrates and fats for energy, less is available for fetus; carrying extra weight is also tiring.

4 Keep them warm, feed them, change their nappies, monitor health, sleep, etc.

10 Human growth and development

10.1 Human growth and development

1 Growth rate is highest at about 6 months to 1 year at over 200 mm per year, it decreases rapidly to 3 years and then levels off / falls slowly until about 11 years, when there is a rapid increase to 100 mm per year at age 14, when the rate falls rapidly to age 19.5–20.

2
a An individual may have a below or above average growth rate.
b The growth spurt for boys may occur later than for girls; this is not shown on the graph.

3 Tables showing growth rate by age and gender

4 Ranges of growth rate for each age / gender

5 Intermediate readings for growth rate or age / separate lines for boys and girls

6 A scatter graph

10.2 Menstrual cycle

1 FSH is inhibited and no new follicles develop; no follicle, no egg, no fertilisation

2 Progesterone

3 FSH and LH

4 Around day 14 of a 28-day cycle

5 Advantages: both allow some couples to have children, increase chances of a live embryo as several eggs collected, can reduce risk of genetic disorder due to embryo selection, by-passes blocked oviduct.
Disadvantages: cost and safety, may be other reasons why woman cannot have a baby.
IVM: less costly than IVF, safer for women who might have side effects from hormone treatment, shorter treatment time.

11 Inheritance and genetic engineering

11.1 Inheritance

1 Both parents are Rr. The son could be Rr or RR, the daughter is rr. The probability of a third child being able to roll its tongue is 3:1 or 75% or 3 out of 4. The chances of a son or daughter are 1:1 or 50:50 or 50%.

2 The father. 50% of the sperm carry the X chromosome, 50% the Y chromosome. All eggs carry the X chromosome.

3 The gene for haemophilia is carried on the X chromosome. Boys inherit the X chromosome from their mother. A carrier mother can pass the gene to her son. She can also pass the gene to a daughter, if the father has haemophilia he will also pass the gene to his daughter; she will be homozygous and have haemophilia.

11.2 Genetic engineering

1 Quick, relatively cheap, no use of animals, dead bodies, urine, blood; identical to human proteins.

2 Oxygen and sugar for energy to build protein, supply of amino acids for making protein, suitable temperature, pH. Other nutrients and a method of removing carbon dioxide also required.

3 Pros: healthy child born, faulty gene not passed to next generation.
Cons: may be risky for embryo, we don't know what future problems may arise, is it ethical?

4 There would be a ready supply of stem cells. The cells would not be rejected.

12 Pathogens and defence against disease

12.1 Pathogens and disease

1

a Bacteria in dirty water and lack of adequate water and sanitation in the capital.

b People who travelled carried the bacteria in their faeces and may have contaminated the water.

c Babies and the elderly.

d Lack of clean water, poor sanitation, overcrowding, lack of medical facilities e.g. medicines. People move about freely from the overcrowded capital to the provinces.

e Boil all drinking water. Wash hands thoroughly in boiled water before handling food. Cover food to prevent flies moving from contaminated water to food. Wash hands after passing faeces. Prevent contamination of water supplies by faeces.

f Vaccination.

2 The bacteria, which stop the thrush developing, are killed by antibiotics along with the disease causing bacteria.

3

a Spray insecticide, use insect repellents on the skin, use a net covering when in bed, try to keep malaria sufferers away from mosquitoes.

b Wash food thoroughly in contaminated areas, boil water for drinking, wash hands thoroughly when preparing food.

4

a Cover nose / mouth with tissues. Flush tissues away. Avoid crowded rooms. Wash hands regularly.

b Always wash hands thoroughly, especially after visiting toilet. Wear clean aprons / overalls. Keep food covered. Keep food cool. If infected, do not handle food at all.

12.2 Defence against disease

1 The plate would be covered. The lid would be taped on. The plate would be in an incubator.

2 He had studied bacteria and knew they should grow unless something was stopping them.

3 They read Fleming's research paper. There were several people, with different scientific knowledge, working together. They selected the best mould. They tested large numbers of infected mice. They received research grants to find out more. They tested the drug on people. They may have had better equipment ten years after Fleming's work.

4 For example, using mice which have been deliberately infected with bacteria; testing a man when too little penicillin was available to finish his treatment.

5 Viruses live inside body cells. To reach them the cells would also be destroyed. Antibiotics are specifically made to target bacteria.

12.3

1 The list should include anything which may lead to cross contamination between equipment, people and the ward surroundings. It will include coughing, sneezing and personal contact.

2 The advice should relate to the following ideas: hand hygiene, cleaning, disinfection and sterilisation of wards and equipment; wearing personal protective equipment such as masks and surgical gloves; preventing infection by vaccination of hospital workers; monitoring, treating and possibly isolating staff / patients after contact with severe infection; being watchful for an infection outbreak.

13 The immune response

13.1 The immune response

1 The antibodies fit the antigens on virus A; they do not match those on B.

2 The cold and 'flu viruses mutate, this changes the antigens and the antibodies cannot recognise them. New lymphocytes must multiply to produce the correct antibodies.

3 The antibodies can work immediately, e.g. destroy the rabies.

4 The primary response is slower and there are less antibodies at the peak.

5 He had used previous knowledge and good observations to form his hypothesis. He took some risks with young children during testing. He had insufficient evidence to prove his hypothesis. Eventually he had more evidence. His treatment seemed to work and no-one died.

6

a The vaccine must be safe before trials with humans.

b The side effects could be widespread.

7 It takes time to produce eggs. If hens die in a bird flu epidemic the eggs will not be available.

🅐 Cancer

14.1 Cancer

1 Eat a healthy, well balanced diet with adequate fibre. Avoid too much ultraviolet light. Have the HPV vaccine. Do not smoke. Monitor moles for changes.

2 To act as a baseline for comparison.

3 No, there is a range of causes for most cancers. If no one smoked there would be 90% less deaths from lung cancer – millions every year.

4 If a few cells are left they can grow into another tumour. Cells might enter the bloodstream and cause a secondary tumour.

5 The more cigarettes smoked, the higher the number of deaths from lung cancer.

Cigarette smoking increased to a maximum in about 1952.
The number of lung cancer deaths increased between 1920 and 1980.
The number of deaths started to fall around 1972.
Cancer deaths occur about 20 years after smoking started.

🅑 21st century health

15.1 21st century health

1 There are many possible suggestions, but basically they should reduce fat and carbohydrate intake, increase fruit and vegetables, increase exercise, reduce / don't start drinking alcohol.

2 The general health of the patient – is one nearer to death, will either patient benefit from other treatments, which patient has the closest tissue match? Issues such as cost, age, gender, home responsibilities, status of patient should not influence medical decisions.

3 **For:** Alcohol may taste nice and complement a meal. Drinking is a pleasant social activity. Small amounts of red wine may protect against heart disease.
Against: It slows reactions, people may become aggressive, binge drinking can make you ill or kill you, long term damage to brain, liver, pancreas and other organs, increased risk of some cancers and diabetes.

4 Here are some suggestions – there will be others.

The son	His parents	The doctor	The government	The food industry
Responsible for what he eats and his exercise levels	Can encourage healthy eating and give opportunities to exercise	Can diagnose health problems, offer solutions	Can promote healthy eating, can provide exercise facilities	Can ensure ready-made meals have less fat, salt and sugar in them and ensure that foods are accurately labelled

5 Use three large groups of people with known cholesterol levels. One group is given regular garlic, a second group has statins, a third group is given a placebo. After a set period of time, check blood cholesterol. You could refine this by selecting people of a similar age, similar cholesterol levels at start, same gender. Use the same laboratory to conduct the cholesterol test.

Glossary

A

accuracy: an accurate measurement is close to the true value.

ADH: *see* antidiuretic hormone.

adolescence: the teenage years when there are physical, psychological, behavioural and emotional changes in a person.

adrenaline: hormone produced by adrenal gland.

aerobic respiration: release of energy from food when oxygen is present.

allele: a version of a particular gene.

amylase: enzyme which digests starch.

anaemia: condition caused by lack of iron.

anaerobic respiration: release of energy from food in the absence of oxygen.

angina: pain felt when flow restricted in coronary arteries.

anorexia: condition caused by extreme dieting due to negative self image.

antagonistic: working in opposite directions.

antibiotics: chemicals produced by fungi which can kill bacteria.

antibodies: produced by white cells to attack antigens.

antidiuretic hormone (ADH): hormone which reduces loss of water in urine.

antigens: foreign chemicals, including protein, which trigger an immune response.

antiseptics: chemicals used to kill pathogens outside the body.

anti-toxins: chemicals produced by the body to counteract toxins (poisons).

artery: blood vessel which carries blood away from the heart.

assimilation: the way the body uses digested food.

atrium (pl. atria): upper chamber in heart.

B

blood: transport medium containing cells and plasma.

C

capillaries: minute blood vessels which form a network close to cells.

carbohydrase: enzyme which digests carbohydrate.

carbohydrate: sugar-based food providing energy.

carcinogen: chemicals which cause cancer.

cartilage: smooth tissue which covers ends of bones.

catalyst: speeds up a chemical reaction.

cataract: clouding of the eye lens.

cell: basic unit of the body.

cell surface membrane: surrounds cytoplasm and controls movement of materials in and out of the cell.

chemotherapy: treament using drugs.

chromosomes: threads of genetic material in the nucleus.

cilia: tiny hair-like structures on surface of cells of airways.

ciliary muscles: muscles which alter the shape of the eye lens for focusing.

clones: genetically identical cells.

clotting: process where blood cells are trapped in fibrin to form a clot.

clumping: process when red cells stick together, not to be confused with clotting.

coeliac disease: a condition where the immune system attacks gut lining, triggered by gluten.

constrict: closing up or getting narrower.

contraception: methods to prevent sperm reaching an egg or prevent implantation.

cornea: clear covering on eye.

coronary artery: artery that supplies heart muscle.

cystic fibrosis: a genetic disorder where the person produces very sticky mucus.

cytoplasm: region of cell in which most chemical reactions take place.

D

data: a collection of measurements.

deamination: breakdown of surplus amino acids to form urea.

denatured: altered shape of an enzyme so it cannot work.

diabetes: condition resulting in high blood sugar if not controlled.

dialysis tubing: a partially permeable membrane used in dialysis machines.

differentiation: the process by which stem cells change to specialised cells.

diffusion: net movement of particles (solute or gas) from a region of high concentration to a region of low concentration.

digestive juice: juices containing enzymes, produced by digestive system.

dilate: open up or get wider.

DNA: deoxyribose nucleic acid, the chemical which carries the genetic code.

dominant: the characteristic which is shown when two different alleles are present.

donor: the person who gives blood or an organ for transplant.

E

effectors: muscles or glands which respond to stimuli.

egestion: removal of waste from the rectum.

egg: female sex cell.

emulsification: breakdown of fat into droplets.

endocrine glands: glands which secrete hormones directly into the bloodstream.

enzyme: a biological catalyst made of protein.

epiglottis: flap which covers opening of trachea (windpipe) when swallowing.

errors: cause readings to be different from the true value.

exchange surface: any surface which allows substances to pass between the blood and cells or blood and the outside.

excretion: removal of waste materials produced by the cells.

F

fair test: only the independent variable affects the dependent variable, other variables are controlled.

fibre: insoluble food material found in vegetables.

fibrin: insoluble fibres which form a clot.

fibrinogen: a soluble blood protein which changes to fibrin in clotting.

fracture: damage to bones.

FSH: follicle stimulating hormone produced by the pituitary.

G

gametes: sex cells.

gene: a section of DNA which codes for the production of a protein.

genotype: the genes present to control a characteristic.

glucagon: hormone produced by pancreas which causes an increase in blood sugar.

glucose: a simple sugar, the most common energy source used in respiration.

glycogen: an insoluble carbohydrate made from glucose molecules.

H

haemodialysis: treatment of blood in dialysis machines.

haemoglobin: protein and iron compound which carries oxygen.

heterozygous: the person has two different alleles for a characteristic, e.g. Aa.

homeostasis: the process by which the body maintains a constant internal environment.

homozygous: the person has two identical alleles for a characteristic, e.g. aa or AA.

hormone: a chemical messenger produced by endocrine glands.

hypothalamus: region of brain containing temperature and pressure receptors.

I

insulin: hormone produced by pancreas which causes a reduction in blood sugar.

ion: a charged atom, e.g. chloride.

K

keyhole surgery: operations where very tiny incisions are made.

L

lactic acid: chemical produced in anaerobic respiration.

lens: focuses light onto the retina.

LH: luteinising hormone produced by the pituitary.

ligaments: strong bands of connective tissue which hold bones together.

lipase: enzyme which digests lipids (fats).

lipid: fat-based food used for insulation and energy storage.

lymphocyte: white blood cell which produces antibodies.

M

malnutrition: too much or too little food or lack of one or more essential nutrients.

meiosis: cell division which halves the number of chromosomes to make gametes.

metabolism: the chemical reactions which take place in the body.

microvilli: folds on cells on surface of villi.

mineral: essential inorganic compounds needed for healthy growth, e.g. sodium chloride.

mitochondria: cell structures which release energy in aerobic respiration.

mitosis: cell division which produces two identical cells.

molecule: two or more atoms joined together, e.g. carbon dioxide, protein.

motor nerves: nerves which carry impulses from the central nervous system to effectors.

mucus: fluid produced by cells to lubricate body tubes.

mutation: spontaneous change in a gene or chromosome.

N

nucleus: cell structure containing chromosomes and controls cell activities.

nutritional information: information about content of food.

O

oesophagus: the gullet, the pipe which carries food from mouth to stomach.

oestrogen: hormone produced by ovary.

organ: a structure made from several tissues with a particular function, e.g. heart.

osmoregulation: control of water.

osmosis: net movement of water from a region of high water concentration to low water concentration.

osteoarthritis: a condition where the joint cartilage is damaged resulting in pain and lack of movement.

osteoporosis: a condition where the bone mass is reduced.

ovulation: release of egg from the ovary.

P

pancreas: gland which produces insulin, glucagon and digestive enzymes.

partially permeable: allows selected substances through.

pathogens: organisms which cause disease.

peristalsis: waves of muscle contraction.

phagocyte: white blood cell which engulfs pathogens.

phenotype: the physical appearance of a characteristic.

pituitary: endocrine gland at base of brain.

placenta: barrier between blood of mother and fetus which allows materials to diffuse across.

plaque: sticky layer on teeth containing bacteria.

plasma: the liquid part of the blood.

plasmid: ring of DNA found in bacteria.

platelets: cell fragments in blood needed for clotting.

posture: the position of the body.

precision: determined by the limits of the scale on the instrument used for a measurement; precise measurements have very little spread around the mean value.

progesterone: hormone produced by ovary.

protease: enzyme which digests protein.

protein: food used for growth and repair.

puberty: the age when the secondary sexual characteristics develop.

Punnett square : a genetic diagram to illustrate crosses.

R

radiotherapy: treament using radiation.

receptors: structures which detect stimuli.

recessive: a characteristic which is masked when the dominant allele is present.

recipient: the person who receives blood or organ.

red blood cell: blood cell containing haemoglobin.

reflex action: an automatic response to a stimulus.

reliability: reliable results can be repeated by someone else.

respiration: release of energy from food.

retina: contains light sensitive cells.

ribosomes: cell structures which make protein.

rickets: condition caused by lack of vitamin D.

S

saliva: alkaline fluid containing amylase.

salivary glands: glands in cheek and under tongue.

scurvy: condition caused by lack of vitamin C.

sense organs: organs which contain receptor cells to detect external stimuli.

sensory nerves: nerves which carry impulses from receptors to the central nervous system.

sex-linked gene: the gene is situated on the X chromosome.

solute: a substance which dissolves in water.

sperm: male sex cell.

sprain: damage to ligaments.

starvation: lack of food.

strains: damage to muscles.

suspensory ligaments: small 'strings' which are attached to the eye lens.

synovial fluid: a fluid which lubricates joints and reduces friction.

synovial joint: joints which contain synovial fluid and can move easily.

system: a group of organs with a shared function, e.g. circulatory system.

T

tendon: joins muscle to bone.

testosterone: hormone produced by testis.

thermoregulation: control of temperature.

thryoxin: hormone produced by thyroid gland which controls metabolic rate.

thyroid: endocrine gland in neck.

tissue: a group of similar cells.

toxins: poisonous substances.

transfusion: transfer of blood or blood products to a patient.

transplant: transfer of organs or tissues from donor to recipient.

true value: this is the value you would obtain if the quantitiy could be measured without any errors at all.

tumour: an abnormal growth of cells.

U

urea: chemical made from excess amino acids found in urine.

urine: solution of urea, salts and other compounds.

V

validity: data is valid if the measurements are only affected by the independent variable and there is no observer bias.

valves: flaps to prevent backflow in circulation.

vector: a carrier of disease-causing organisms.

veins: blood vessels which carry blood to the heart.

ventricle: lower chamber in heart.

villi: folds on surface of gut lining.

vitamin: nutrient needed in small quantities for healthy growth.

voluntary action: an action which involves thinking by the brain.

W

white blood cell: blood cell of the immune system.

Z

zygote: the first cell produced when the sperm fertilises the egg.

Index

Key terms are in bold.

A

absorption 23
active immunity 97
acupuncture 106
ADH *see* antidiuretic hormone
adolescence 74
adrenal glands 54, 55
adrenaline 54, 55
aerobic respiration 11
alcohol 105, 107
  breath tests 48
  pregnancy 73
alkaline salts 23
alleles 79, 81
'alternative' therapies 106–7
alveoli 34, 35, 36
Alzheimer's disease 53
amnion 72
amniotic fluid 72
amoebic dysentery 85
amylase 21
anaemia 16, 27
anaerobic respiration 11
anaesthesia 59
angina 31
anorexia 16
antagonistic muscle pairs 61
antibiotics 85, 90, 99
  cholera 86
  discovery 88
  penicillin 88
  resistance 89
antibodies 87, 96
  vaccines 97, 99
antidiuretic hormone (ADH) 57
antigens 27, 96
  see also immune response
antiseptics 90, 99
anti-toxins 87
arteries 28, 29, 30
arthritis 62 *see also* osteoarthritis

artificial immunity 97
artificial lungs 36
assimilation 24
atheroma 30, 31
Athlete's foot 85
atria 29

B

bacteria 84
  cholera 86
  genetic engineering 82
  infection treatment 85
  large intestine 25
Banting, Frederick G. 55, 56
Barnard, Christiaan 32
benign tumours 100
Best, Charles H. 55, 56
bile 23
birth 70, 72–3, 75
blood 26–33, 83, 87
  artificial lungs 36
  circulation 26, 28–33
  excretion 49
  groups 27
  hormones 54–8
  red cells 26, 60
  sugar levels 55–8
  white cells 26, 60, 87, 96–7
body temperature 58–9
bones 60, 61
  leukaemia 83
  skeletal health 62, 63
brain 35, 50, 100

C

cancer 83, 100–3
capillaries 28, 29
carbohydrases 20
carbohydrates 14, 15, 20
carcinogens 101
cardiac physiologists 31
cardiographers 31
cartilage 61, 62

catalysts 13
cataracts 53
cells 10
  division 78
  organisation 11
  processes 12–13
  respiration 11
cell surface membranes 10
central nervous system (CNS) 50
CF *see* cystic fibrosis
Chain, Ernst 88
chemical code 79
chemotherapy 102
chiropractors 62
cholera 86
chromosomes 71, 78, 81
cilia 34, 52, 87
ciliary muscles 52
circulation 26, 28–33
clones 82, 83
close contact transmission 86
Clostridium difficile 90
clotting 26, 87
clumping 27
CNS *see* central nervous system
coeliac disease 25
cold receptors 59
competition 89, 90
contraception 75
coordination 50, 54–7
corneas 52
coronary arteries 30
counsellors 79
cystic fibrosis (CF) 25
  genetic counsellors 79, 80
  testing 81
cytologists 10
cytoplasm 10
cytotechnologists 10

D

deamination 24
dehydration 58

denaturation   13
deoxygenated blood   28
deoxyribose nucleic acid, *see* DNA
diabetes   16, 55
diagnosing cancer   101
dialysis   47, 48
diaphragm   34
diet   14–17, 105
dieting   16–17
differentiation   83
diffusion   12, 72
digestion   20–5, 22
discs   61, 62
disease   84
dislocation   62
DNA   81
   genetic engineering   83
   inheritance   78
   viruses   84
Doll, Richard   102
dominant alleles   79
donors   27, 48
double circulation   28
drinking habits   105
droplet infections   86
drug habits   106
dysentery   85

E

eating habits   105
   see also diet
economics   104
effector cells   51
egestion   25
egg   70
embryos   71
emulsification   23
endocrine glands   54, 55
endocrinologists   54
energy   11
engulfment   96
Entamoeba histolytica   85
enzymes   13, 24
   denaturation   13
   food breakdown   20

genetic engineering   82, 83
   optimum function   13
   pH   13, 22
epidemics   86, 89
epiglottis   21
ethics   104
exchange surfaces   29
excretion   46–9, 48
exercise   105
eyes   52–3

F

fat   14, 15, 16, 20, 23
feedback systems   57, 76
female reproductive system   70
fertilisation   71, 72
fertility   75, 76
fetal alcohol syndrome   105
fetus   71, 105
fibre   14, 15
fibrin   26
fibrinogen   26
Fleming, Alexander   88
Florey, Howard   88
follicle stimulating hormone (FSH)   54, 55, 76, 77
food   18–19
   see also digestion; nutrition
fractures   62
fraternal twins   72
FSH *see* follicle stimulating hormone
fungi   84, 85

G

gall bladder   23
gametes   71
gas exchange   34–6
genes   78, 79, 82
gene therapy   82
genetic counsellors   79, 80
genetic engineering   78, 82–3
genotypes   79
ginseng   107
glucagon   54, 55, 56
glucose   11, 55, 56, 57
glycogen   11

growth   74–5
gut   22

H

haemodialysis   47, 48
haemoglobin   26
health   104–7
   see also cancer; diet; nutrition
heart
   circulation   28, 29, 30–1
   muscle   30–1
   transplants   32
'heart–lung' machines   32
heat receptors   59
herbal medicine   106–7
heterozygous genotypes   79
homeopathy   106
homeostasis   58–9, 58
homozygous genotypes   79
hormones   50, 54, 55–7
   growth/puberty   74–5
   menstrual cycles   76–7
hospital infection control   89
Huntington's disease   79, 80
hyperthermia   59
hypothalamus   57, 59, 75

I

identical twins   72
immune response   96–9
immunological memory   96
infection   84, 86, 89
infectious diseases   84
infertility treatments   76
influenza   99
inheritance   78–81
insulin   54, 55
   diabetes   55, 56, 57
   genetic engineering   82
   production   56
intercostal muscles   34
internal defences   87
ions   12
islets   56

J

Jenner, Edward 98
joints 60, 61, 62–3

K

keyhole surgery 63
kidneys 46, 48

L

labelling food 18–19
labour 73
lactic acid 11
large intestine 25
lenses 52
leukaemia 83
LH *see* luteinizing hormone
life expectancy 104
ligaments 61
light 51, 52, 53, 101
lipases 20
lipids 14, 15, 16, 20, 23
liver 23, 24, 46
living organ transplants 32
long sightedness 53
lungs 32, 34, 36
luteinizing hormone (LH) 55, 76, 77
lymphocytes 26, 96, 97
lymph system 26, 96, 97, 100, 101

M

malaria 85
male reproductive system 70
malignant tumours 100
malnutrition 16
medicine 106–7
meiosis 71, 78
menstrual cycles 72, 74, 76–7
microbes 84
microbiologists 89
microvilli 24
mind therapies 106
minerals 14, 15, 16
mitochondria 10
mitosis 71, 78
molecules 12

mosquitoes 85
motor nerves 50
movement 60–1
mucus 21
muscle 60, 61
   eyes 52
   heart 30–1
mutations 78, 79, 89

N

natural immunity 96
natural selection 89
negative feedback systems 57, 76
nerves 50
nervous system 50–3
neurones 50
nucleus 10
nutrients 11, 15
nutrition 14–19, 18, 105

O

oesophagus 21
oestrogen 54, 55
   growth/puberty 74, 75
   menstrual cycles 76, 77
optimum temperatures 13
optometrists 53
organs 11, 32
organ transplants 32
osmoregulation 59
osmosis 12, 12
osteoarthritis 62
osteopaths 62
osteoporosis 62
OTC *see* over-the-counter drug habits
outbreaks 89–90
outer defences 87
over-the-counter (OTC) drug habits 106
oviducts 72
ovulation 72, 74
oxygen 11, 28
   see also respiration

P

pacemakers 31
pancreas 22, 23, 54, 55

pandemics 89
partial permeability 12
passive immunity 97
pasteurisation 86
pathogens 84–90, 84
   see also bacteria; immune response
penicillin 88
peristalsis 22
peritoneal dialysis 47, 48
permeability 12
pH 22, 35
phagocytes 26, 96
phenotypes 79
physiotherapists 62
pituitary glands 75
placenta 72
plaque 20
plasma 26
plasmids 82, 83
platelets 26
posture 61, 62
precautionary protective mechanisms 87
pressure 30, 34
progesterone 54, 55
   menstrual cycles 76, 77
proteases 20
protection 60
   against disease 87
   organs 60
proteins 14, 15, 20
protoctistans 84, 85
puberty 74–5, 74
Punnett squares 80–1, 80

R

radiotherapy 102
RDAs *see* recommended daily amounts
receptor cells 35, 51, 58, 59
recessive alleles 79
recommended daily amounts (RDAs) 14
red blood cells 26, 60
reflex actions 50, 51
relay neurones 50

reproduction 70–3, 90
resistance 89–90
respiration 11, 35, 36
retina 52
ribonucleic acid (RNA) 84
ribosomes 10, 13
ribs 34
rickets 16
RNA 84

S

saliva 21, 49
salivary glands 21
scabs 87
scurvy 16
secondary tumours 101
selection 89, 90
sense organs 52
sensory nerves 50
sensory neurones 51
sex cells 71
sex-linked genes 81
short sightedness 53
skeleton 60, 61, 62–3
skin 58, 87
small intestine 23
smallpox 98
smoking
  bone cells 63
  cancer 101, 102, 103
  pregnancy 73
  see also cancer
solutes 12
sperm 70, 79
sprains 62
starvation 16
statin 106

stem cells 33, 71, 83
stomach 23
strains 62
strokes 31
substrate 24
sugar 55, 56, 57
support 60
surface areas 20
survival 89, 90
suspensory ligaments 52
swallowing 21
sweating 58
synapses 51
synovial fluid 61
systems 11

T

target organs 54
teeth 21
tendons 61, 62
testing food 18–19
testosterone 54, 55
  growth/puberty 74, 75
therapies 83, 106–7
thermoregulation 58, 59
thyroid 54, 55
tidal volume 35
tissues 11
touch 51
toxins 47, 87
trachea 34
transfusions 27
transplants 32, 48
treating cancer 102
tumours 100
twenty-first century health 104–7
twins 72

U

ultraviolet light 101
universal donors 27
urea 24, 25, 46
urine 46, 49
uterus 72–3

V

vaccines 96, 97, 98–9
valves 29
vectors 85, 86
veins 28, 29
ventricles 29
villi 23, 24
viruses 84, 86
vital capacities 35
vitamins 14, 15, 16
volume 34, 35
voluntary actions 50

W

warfarin 107
water 47, 57, 58
  see also osmosis
white blood cells 26
  lymphocytes 96
  pathogen destruction 87
  production 60
  vaccines 97

Z

zygotes 71, 78

Acknowledgements

Photo acknowledgements

The author and publisher are grateful to the following for permission to reproduce photographs and other copyright material in this book.

Alamy: Owe Andersson / 04.01D; Peter Arnold, Inc. / 11.01A; Chapter 12 Opener; 12.01D; Gregory Bergman / 15.01E; Biodisc/Visuals Unlimited / Chapter 6 Opener; Caro / 07.02D; Adrian Davies / 08.02C; Shaun Finch - Coyote-Photography.co.uk / 02.02Ac; Garry Gay / Chapter 15 Opener; David Gregs / Chapter 9 Opener; JUPITERIMAGES/Polka Dot / 07.04A; Jonathon Laming / Chapter 8 Opener; Medical-on-Line / 12.01C; MedicalRF.com / Chapter 14 Opener; Photodisc / Chapter 2 Opener; Photononstop / 02.01B; PhotoStock-Israel / 15.01D; PHOTOTAKE Inc. / Chapter 10 Opener; Chapter 11 Opener; 11.01B; 12.02B; Picture Press / 15.01F; Powered by Light RF / 02.02Ab; Science Photo Library / Chapter 7 Opener; Shout / 09.02C; Stephen Sweet / 09.01B; Janine Wiedel Photolibrary / 11.01H; **Food Standards Agency**: /02.01A (Crown copyright material is reproduced with the permission from the controller, Office of Public Sector Information (OPSI); **Fotolia:** Dmitry Knorre / 12.01E; Moose408 / Chapter 16 Opener; **istockphoto.com**: Jani Bryson / 15.01C; Tom England / 02.02Aa; 14.01D; Andy Green / 02.01Ga; Sven Hoppe / 10.01C; Christine Kublanski / 06.01D; Timothy Large / 05.01E; Phil Pell/14.01E; **Science Photo Library:** AJ Photo / 04.02I; Dr Klaus Boller / Chapter 13 Opener; Dee Breger / 08.02D; CNRI / 03.01B; 05.01F; Eye of Science / 03.02E; Chapter 3 Opener; 05.01G; 08.02E; Mauro Fermariello / 01.01B; Steve Gschmeissner / Chapter 1 Opener; 03.02F; 03.02G; Gustoimages / 14.01B; John Heseltine / 02.01Gb; Hossler, Custom Medical Stock Photo / Chapter Opener 5; Andrew Lambert Photography / 02.02B; Professors P. M. Motta and F. M. Magliocca / 03.02H; D Phillips / 12.03C; Prof. Aaron Polliack / Chapter 4 Opener; 04.01B; Antonia Reeve / 04.02J; Science Photo Library / 04.02G; 07.03C; Dr Linda Stannard, UCT / 12.01A; St Mary's Hospital Medical School / 12.02A; Jim Varney / 12.03B.

Every effort has been made to trace and contact all copyright holders and we apologise if any have been overlooked. The publisher will be pleased to make the necessary arrangements at the first opportunity.